Interceptive orthodontics

Fourth edition

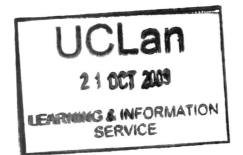

Interceptive orthodontics

Fourth edition

Andrew Richardson, MSc, BDS, DPD, FFD, DOrth

Emeritus Professor of Orthodontics, The Queens University of Belfast
Consultant, The Royal Group of Hospitals and Dental Hospital, Belfast

1999

Published by the British Dental Association
64 Wimpole Street, London W1M 8AL

This book is dedicated to my wife, Margaret who claims to have
deterred me from flights of fancy while it was being written and
who dissociates herself from some of the statements made
therein, and to my friends and colleagues without whose constant
interest, support and constructive criticism it would have been
completed in half the time.

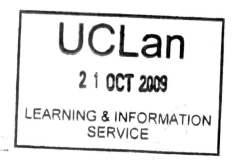
First edition   1982
Second edition   1989
Third edition   1995
Fourth edition   1999

ISBN 0 904588 56 4

Printed and bound by Dennis Barber Graphics and Print,
Lowestoft, Suffolk

Contents

'Yes', said Bond. He looked levelly at the great red face across the desk. 'It's a remarkable case history. Galloping paranoia. Delusions of jealousy and persecution. Megalomaniac hatred and desire for revenge. Curiously enough', he went on conversationally, 'it may have something to do with your teeth. Diastema they call it. Comes from sucking your thumb when you're a child. Yes, I expect that's what the psychologists will say when they get you into the lunatic asylum. "Ogre's teeth." Being bullied at school and so on. Extraordinary the effect it has on a child.'

Ian Fleming, *'Moonraker'*

Preface to the fourth edition

Seventeen years ago, when the first edition of this book was published, there were few dentists with an orthodontic qualification and most orthodontic work in Britain was carried out by enthusiastic general practitioners. This was the target group for the pocket-sized first edition.

Today, there are more orthodontists and more orthodontically-aware practitioners as a result of improved undergraduate education and extended and more formalised postgraduate training.

Improvements in the quantity and quality of communication in all its forms has ensured that dentists know more, orthodontists know more, and patients know and expect more. The reduction in dental caries has brought about a shift in emphasis from dental comfort to dental aesthetics, and with it a greater tolerance for fixed appliances. Fixed appliances are more readily available because of improvements in dental materials, the advent of preformed components and diminishing costs from competition between the supply houses.

There is nobody more enthusiastic about fixed appliances than I am. It is interesting, challenging, precise and fulfilling work. However, I see around me the shortcomings of fixed-appliances in terms of inexpert handling, poor compliance, loss of anchorage, relapse and iatrogenic root resorption, decalcification and periodontal breakdown.

Against this background, interceptive orthodontics must have an important place in modern orthodontic practice, not necessarily as an alternative, but alongside mechanical treatment. Patients who have grown accustomed to the concept of crooked teeth needing braces may be surprised to be told that they might not need braces at all. They must feel that they have attended a kind of faith healer, a witch doctor who will charm away their malocclusion or any other ailment they care to mention. Interception is not like that. It has its limitations. It is quite restricted in its applicability and the timing of interceptive treatment is crucial.

Previous editions of this book have been criticised for being insufficiently didactic and dogmatic. I took that as a compliment. On the other hand, if all of the exceptions to the general rules were recognised in the body of a text, it would be very confusing and overly scientific. Dogma is attractive because it is easy to teach and easy to learn but Dentistry is moving away from the dogma taught by experienced teachers whose opinions have perhaps been clouded by their most recent successful (or unsuccessful) case. The concepts of peer review, audit and evidence-based dentistry are with us. However, if this textbook were based exclusively on evidence meeting modern criteria for high quality research, it would be quite small. Research techniques appropriate to clinical trials may not be applicable in orthodontics much of which is related to infinite variations in growth and it is impossible to stop growth in a control group. The implications are that studies should be longitudinal and the samples must be large. Likewise, I have reservations regarding the fashionable meta-analysis on account of variations in the quality of records and the reproducibility of cephalometric measurements.

These conflicting considerations make it difficult to write a book for the new millennium. In striking a compromise, I have been guided by a quotation from Asbjørn Jokstad:[1] 'Evidence-based dentistry is much more than randomised controlled trials and must always be regarded as an adjunct to, and not a substitute for, sound clinical judgement and patient preferences.' As before, I have tried to present a coherent, comprehensible story line in each chapter which represents the consensus opinion but at the end of each chapter, under the heading of 'Summary of evidence' I have given brief factual summaries of the more robust and respected research work on the subject. These may relieve practitioners of the physical labour involved in hunting out papers and make it easier for them to make their own assessments of what the evidence shows.[2,3] The summaries should also make the book more relevant to the orthodontist and trainee orthodontist.

This fourth edition, like its predecessors, is intended for anyone who cares to read it. Previous editions have proved popular with undergraduate students and those in vocational training along with dentists, rather than orthodontists, in all spheres of dentistry round the world. Bearing this in mind, I have tried to maintain a simplicity and economy of style while incorporating updated material. Almost all chapters have been altered in this way, but the most significant addition is a new chapter on screening the child community for interception and the outcome of interceptive treatment. This project was the foundation for a successful PhD thesis by Kazem Al Nimri and I am grateful to him for the part he played in the project. As always, I am grateful to Mike Grace, Stephen Hancocks and the staff of the British Dental Journal and BDA Information Centre for their help and forbearance. I am grateful to Sheena Sloan and the staff of the Department of Medical Photography at the Royal Group of Hospitals for preparing the illustrations and to Gordon Douglas who made the models and appliances. Jim Moss very kindly read the script and made many useful suggestions, most of which were quickly incorporated into the text. We agreed to differ on a few points – we are orthodontists after all.

I have always seen the orthodontic care of growing, developing and maturing children as a privilege which brings great satisfaction when the aims of treatment are achieved. I hope these thoughts will be expressed between the lines of the pages which follow and that the reader will derive as much pleasure from the practice of orthodontics as I do.

Andrew Richardson
Orthodontic Department
School of Dentistry
Royal Victoria Hospital
Belfast BT12 6BP
1999

References

1 Jokstad A. Evidence-based healthcare: avoiding ivory tower research? *Evidence-based Dentistry* 1998; 1:5–6.
2 Grace, Mike. Evidence-based dentistry. *Br Dent J* 1997; **182**: 323.
3 Grace, Mike. Nothing but the evidence. *Br Dent J* 1998; **184**: 105.

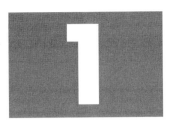

Interception defined — the need for interception

Most orthodontic treatment is carried out for a patient who is constantly growing and developing in a way determined by the inherited genetic constitution interacting with the local environment.

The present emphasis in orthodontics on materials and appliances tends to make orthodontists believe that the success or failure of treatment resides completely in the appliance and encourages them to forget the implications of natural growth changes. It is worth remembering that all an orthodontist can do with an appliance is to change the local environment.

If treatment could be completed within a short space of time, the immediate implications of growth and development would be insignificant, but the fact of the matter is that most orthodontic treatments extend over 18 months or 2 years and spontaneous developmental changes cannot be ignored. In addition, growth changes following completion of treatment may spoil a fine result. No matter how powerful the appliance used, its effects will be more simple, natural and stable if the treatment is in harmony with spontaneous growth and development. It is easier to swim with the tide.

Some spontaneous developmental changes are favourable, others are not. Figure 1.1 shows a patient at age 12 years with the upper incisors in lingual occlusion. Following extraction of lower first premolars, he was treated with removable appliances to procline the upper incisors and retrocline the lower incisors. During treatment, the mandible grew to such an extent that the patient was left with upper incisors still behind the lowers and an anterior open bite. Figure 1.2 shows a patient who presented with proclined and spaced incisors and an anterior open bite. After 6 months, without treatment, the incisors had retroclined and the open bite had closed.[1]

Favourable and unfavourable changes of a more localised nature can also occur. Figure 1.3 shows a distally inclined and apparently impacted lower second premolar which erupted spontaneously. Figure 1.4 shows a third molar which seemed to have sufficient space for eruption but subsequently became impacted.

Interceptive treatment is based upon sharp-eyed detection of small variations round the pattern of normal development. Some of these variations are quite subtle. Other, more pronounced discrepancies may show remarkable powers of spontaneous correction. Thus, decisions on whether interceptive measures are necessary or desirable are often not straightforward. Informed decisions can be based only on sound knowledge and extensive experience of normal occlusal development and the early signs of developing irregularities.

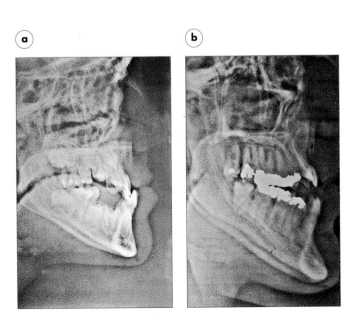

Fig. 1.1 Deterioration during and after orthodontic treatment. (a) age 12 years (b) age 16 years.

There has been much debate over the title which should be given to this aspect of orthodontics. The subject used to be called preventive orthodontics, but the more recent label, interceptive orthodontics, is probably more realistic in terms of clinical possibilities and limitations.

Implicit in the word preventive is the suggestion that the preventive measure can be applied prophylactically before there is any sign or symptom of the anomaly which is to be prevented. The foundations of many malocclusions are laid down at the moment the ovum is fertilised and there is not much that dentistry can do about that. The dentist may not be aware that a malocclusion is developing until some time after the development has started and the irregularity is recognisable clinically or radiologically.

Thus, interception seems the more appropriate term. There are, however, some developing malocclusions which are truly predictable and preventable. One example is secondary crowding in the premolar area subsequent to the extraction of a deciduous molar which is totally predictable and can be prevented by the use of a space maintainer.

There are also some irregularities which can have secondary effects on the developing occlusion. While the presenting malocclusion cannot be prevented until it is seen in the mouth, the secondary malocclusion may be truly preventable.

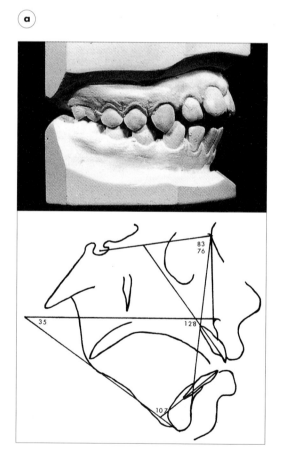
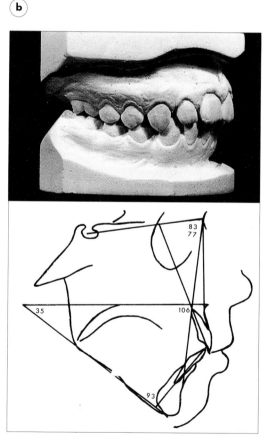

Fig. 1.2 Spontaneous improvement in the incisor relationship. (a) age 16 years (b) 6 months later.

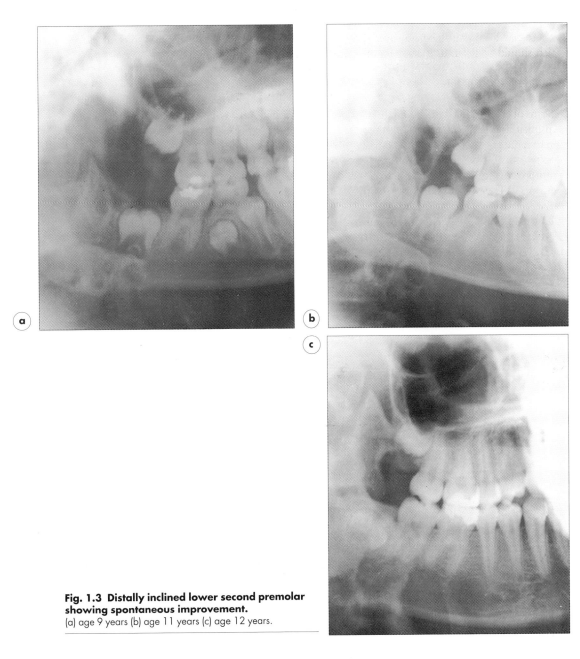

Fig. 1.3 Distally inclined lower second premolar showing spontaneous improvement.
(a) age 9 years (b) age 11 years (c) age 12 years.

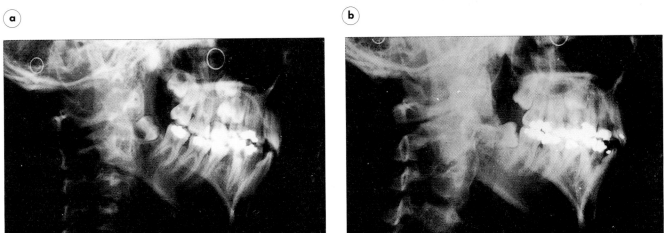

Fig. 1.4 Unpredictable impaction of lower third molar. (a) age 12 years (b) age 17 years.

One example is the upper incisor in lingual occlusion associated with a forward displacement in closing from the rest position. Early correction of the anomalous incisor occlusion will allow the later developing teeth to erupt into the environment of the correct jaw relationship and malocclusion of these teeth may be prevented (Fig. 1.5).

Some authorities make an academic distinction between preventive orthodontics 'any action taken to preserve the integrity of a normal occlusion' and interceptive orthodontics 'procedures that eliminate or reduce the severity of malocclusion'.[2]

Whether these should be called interception, prevention, corrective therapy, guided eruption or early treatment is debatable. What one is interested in doing is fostering developmental changes which are favourable, and halting or minimising those which are not. The last sentence might be taken as a definition of the art or science of interceptive orthodontics.

Mention should be made of another definition of interceptive orthodontics, sometimes called phase 1 treatment or growth modification, during the period of active growth. Some orthodontists apply the term to any treatment in the mixed dentition,[3] others favour early appliance therapy as an optional alternative to treating malocclusions after the permanent dentition is established or as a preliminary phase of treatment.[4]

There should be no conflict between interception and appliance therapy. Ideally, they should be used side by side in orthodontic practice to take the best advantage of both. Sometimes they are alternatives, usually they are not.

Appliance therapy has the advantages of precise positioning of teeth and treating or camouflaging of skeletal discrepancies; interception has the advantage of economy and simplicity without the risks of root resorption, iatrogenic decalcification or periodontal disease. While teeth may move subsequent to interceptive treatment, they will never relapse.

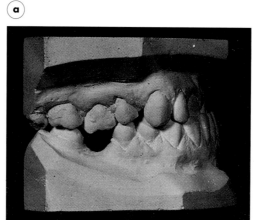
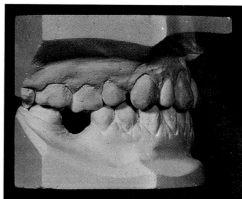

Fig. 1.5 Lingual occlusion of upper incisors with forward displacement. (a) before treatment (b) after treatment. Note the change in occlusal relationship of canines premolars and molars.

References

1 Richardson A. Juliet Bravo: Spontaneous improvement in a patient with Anterior Open Bite. *Br Dent J* 1985; **159**: 256–258.

2 Popovich F, Thompson GW. Evaluation of preventive and interceptive orthodontic treatment between three and eighteen years of age. *Trans Third Int Orthodont Cong* 1973: 260–281.

3 Bass NM. Interceptive Orthodontics. European Orthodontic Society Conference 1996 Abstracts p.10 Keynote address.

4 Woodside DG. Interceptive orthodontics. European Orthodontic Society Conference 1996 Abstracts p.19 Keynote address.

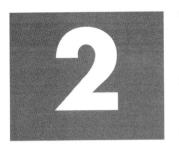

The development of ideal occlusion and the aetiology of malocclusion

The evidence-based findings are summarised on pages 12 and 13.

Occlusal development

Occlusal development occurs in five stages, as shown in Table 2.1.

Edentulous stage

The infant, at birth, has no teeth nor has he any need for teeth. He has instead two tough, firm edentulous arches known as gum pads (Fig. 2.1) The upper gum pad is typically rounded anteriorly, forming a horseshoe shape, whereas the lower is more flattened, making the shape of the letter U.

It is not unusual for the gum pads to be clearly segmented, each segment corresponding to a developing deciduous tooth. The sulcus demarcating the distal edge of the developing deciduous canine is particularly well marked and is carried over on to the buccal side of the pad, where it is known as the lateral sulcus. The relationship of the upper lateral sulcus to the lower is often used to measure the antero-posterior gum pad 'occlusion'.

There has been much debate on the normal or correct relationship of the gum pads and whether the gum pads are ever brought together during life. However, it seems generally agreed that the lower gum pad, at birth, is often posterior to the upper which, in the dentate state, would be regarded as a Class II malocclusion. Also, there is often an oval vertical space anteriorly which, after the eruption of teeth, would be described as an open bite.

Both of these features of the gum pads may be transitory. The postnormality is usually corrected by rapid forward growth of the mandible during the first few months of life, and the vertical space has been considered by some authorities as a favourable feature which may prevent an excessive overbite when the teeth erupt.[1] On the other hand, Leighton[2] found large variations of gum pad relationships in children who subsequently developed normal occlusion, concluding that identification of the normal relationship at the gum pad stage is very difficult.

Eruption of deciduous teeth

The deciduous teeth normally erupt between the ages of 6 months and 2.5 years. The average ages of eruption in Caucasian children[3] are shown in Table 2.2. Males tend to erupt deciduous incisors before females, females tend to erupt deciduous molars and canines before males but the differences are not significant. Eruption in dark-skinned races tends to be earlier than in white Caucasians.

Although most dental students learn the ages of eruption and a typical order of eruption (ABDCE, with the lower erupting before its upper counterpart), the fact of the matter is that variation in the order of eruption and the timing of eruption is the rule rather than the exception. Such variations in the ages of eruption need not give rise to concern unless they are outside the 95% range.

Table 2.1 Stages in the development of occlusion

(Third molar teeth have been excluded because their eruption ages are so variable)

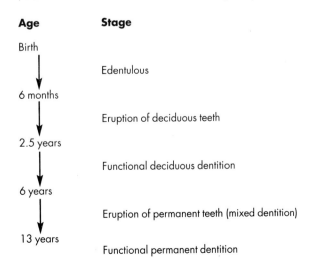

Age	Stage
Birth	
↓	Edentulous
6 months	
↓	Eruption of deciduous teeth
2.5 years	
↓	Functional deciduous dentition
6 years	
↓	Eruption of permanent teeth (mixed dentition)
13 years	
	Functional permanent dentition

Table 2.2 Median (50%) and 5-95% age ranges (months) for eruption of deciduous teeth in female and male Caucasians[3].

Tooth	5%	50%	95%
Upper central	6.8	9.1	12.7
Upper lateral	7.2	9.8	15.0
Upper canine	13.6	17.6	23.8
Upper first molar	11.8	14.8	18.5
Upper second molar	20.1	24.4	26.6
Lower central	4.3	6.8	10.6
Lower lateral	7.9	11.4	16.7
Lower canine	14.0	18.0	24.6
Lower first molar	11.8	15.4	18.8
Lower second molar	20.2	26.2	33.1

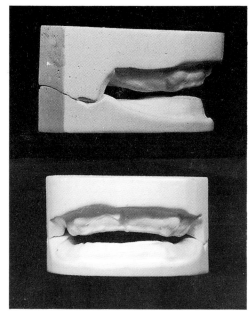

Fig. 2.1 Gum pads shortly after birth.

Functional deciduous dentition

In the fully developed deciduous dentition seen after the age of 2.5 years, the incisor teeth seem very upright and they are usually spaced from each other (Fig. 2.2). These spaces occur most frequently mesial to the upper deciduous canine and distal to the lower deciduous canine. In the monkey family, similar spaces allow for the interdigitation of the long canine teeth and for this reason they are frequently described as anthropoid or primate spaces when they occur in the human. Anthropoid spaces may also occur in the human permanent dentition when the teeth are spaced and the upper canine is often rotated mesio-palatally into the lower anthropoid space.

Concerned mothers often ask whether a spaced deciduous dentition is the forerunner of a gappy permanent set. In the Caucasian, the answer is almost invariably negative. The available evidence indicates that if there is no spacing in the deciduous dentition there is a 70% chance of crowding of the permanent teeth. If there is less than 3mm spacing there is a 50% chance of crowding and it is only when spacing exceeds 6mm that there is little chance of crowding of the permanent teeth.[4] Remarkably, the dental arch length (measured from the labial surfaces of the incisors perpendicular to a line joining the distal surfaces of the second deciduous molars or second premolars) is smaller at 18 years than it is at 3 years.[5] This measurement decreases at about 3 years as spaces between the deciduous molars close, increases at 7-8 years on eruption of the permanent incisors, and decreases again as the deciduous molars are replaced by the premolars.

Ideally, the mesio-buccal cusp of the upper second deciduous molar bites opposite the anterior buccal groove of the lower, which is a similar arrangement to the occlusion of the first molars (the sixes) in the permanent dentition. However, the lower second deciduous molar is such a large tooth that, in the majority of cases, the distal surfaces of the upper and lower second deciduous molars are in the same vertical plane. Should this relationship persist, there will be implications for the occlusion of the first permanent molars when they erupt. In the minority, there is a 'mesial step' with the distal surface of the lower second deciduous molar being mesially placed in relation to the upper.

While an extremely large overbite or overjet in the completed deciduous dentition may indicate a similar arrangement of the permanent successors, lesser variations have a much smaller predictive value.[4]

The overbite shows a sharp increase when the deciduous incisors erupt with a diminution between 2.5 and 7 years due to attrition and some forward translation of the mandible. There is a corresponding increase in the overbite when the permanent incisors erupt with a further increase up to 11 or 12 years. Thereafter, overbites tend to diminish up to the end of the growth period.[6] Open bite of the completed deciduous dentition commonly results from a habit of thumbsucking but, providing the habit is abandoned, the open bite will not be carried through to the permanent teeth.

On the whole, parents do not bring their offspring for treatment of increased overbite and overjet in the deciduous dentition unless the discrepancy is very gross, but they will frequently seek treatment of an anterior or posterior crossbite. The lay person seems much more aware of a chin that sticks out too far or is deviated to one side or to the other. This awareness is fortunate because there is frequently a displacement of the mandible in closing from the rest position in these cases. In general, displacements should be treated early so that occlusal development may proceed on the basis of an undisplaced jaw relationship.

Between the ages of 2.5 and 6 years there is little alteration in the deciduous dentition. The exception is that occlusal attrition may allow forward shift of the mandibular teeth in relation to the maxillary teeth which will be significant when the permanent molars erupt (Fig. 2.3). Although Friel[7] laid great emphasis on this change in the occlusion, the evidence suggests that it occurs in only a minority of cases.[8,9] The uninitiated must be very wary about interpreting this change because young children will frequently protrude the mandible when asked to bring their teeth together.

Eruption of permanent teeth (mixed dentition)

The range of variation in the ages of eruption is remarkable, amounting to 5 years for several teeth. As a general rule, each lower tooth erupts before its counterpart in the upper arch with the exception of the second premolars. There are no significant differences between the ages of eruption of teeth on the left and right sides. In the upper arch, the earliest permanent teeth to erupt are the first permanent molars (the sixes) followed by the central and lateral incisors. The eruption of upper first (and sometimes second) premolars normally precedes eruption of the canines, which should be palpable on the buccal side of the alveolar process after the age of 10 years. In the lower arch the first permanent molars or central incisors may erupt first, usually followed by the lateral incisors, canines, premolars and second molars.[10-15] The age of eruption of permanent teeth is affected by premature loss of deciduous predecessors.[15]

Median and 5%-95% age ranges for eruption (without premature loss of deciduous teeth) in Caucasian females and males are given in Tables 2.3 and 2.4 respectively. The eruption of teeth tends to be earlier in females with the exception of second molars. Teeth which have not erupted within the 95% age limit should be investigated radiologically.

At the age of 6 years, the 'mesial step' in the minority of children allows the first permanent molars to erupt into normal occlusion (Fig. 2.4). However, the majority of children still have the distal surfaces of the second deciduous molars in the same vertical line. In consequence, the first permanent molars often erupt into a cusp-to-cusp relationship in the antero-posterior plane. This relationship is quite common in a dentition which is developing normally and does not necessarily indicate that a Class II malocclusion will ensue.

Table 2.3 Median (50%) and 5–95% age ranges (years) for eruption of permanent teeth in Caucasian females.[15]

Tooth	5%	50%	95%
Upper central	5.99	7.08	7.95
Upper lateral	6.72	8.04	9.49
Upper canine	8.97	10.98	12.79
Upper first premolar	8.50	10.57	12.45
Upper second premolar	9.27	11.32	13.06
Upper first molar	5.60	6.32	7.55
Upper second molar	10.47	12.14	14.15
Lower central	5.56	6.31	7.09
Lower lateral	6.11	7.36	8.68
Lower canine	8.14	9.87	11.41
Lower first premolar	8.64	10.21	11.92
Lower second premolar	9.19	11.34	13.53
Lower first molar	5.53	6.26	7.34
Lower second molar	10.37	11.82	14.15

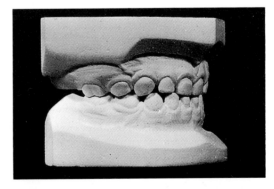

Fig. 2.2 Normal occlusion at age 3 years.

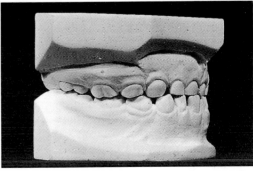

Fig. 2.3 Normal occlusion at age 7 years. Forward movement of the lower arch relative to the upper has facilitated normal interdigitation of the first permanent molars. Same patient as Fig. 2.2

Table 2.4   Median (50%) and 5-95% age ranges (years) for eruption of permanent teeth in Caucasian males.[15]

Tooth	5%	50%	95%
Upper central	6.13	7.12	8.36
Upper lateral	7.26	8.16	9.77
Upper canine	9.64	11.17	13.41
Upper first premolar	8.84	10.66	12.62
Upper second premolar	9.44	11.43	13.62
Upper first molar	5.45	6.39	7.73
Upper second molar	10.30	12.04	13.97
Lower central	5.49	6.23	7.40
Lower lateral	6.29	7.36	8.74
Lower canine	9.00	10.47	13.05
Lower first premolar	8.75	10.52	12.54
Lower second premolar	9.57	11.50	13.48
Lower first molar	5.47	6.31	7.59
Lower second molar	10.04	11.83	13.65

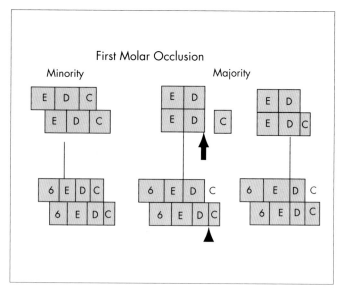

Fig. 2.4 Mechanisms whereby the first permanent molars can achieve a normal relationship. In the minority, the distal surface of the lower second deciduous molar is mesial to the distal surface of the upper, allowing the first permanent molars to erupt into a normal relationship. In the majority, the distal surfaces of the second deciduous molars are in the same vertical plane which makes the first permanent molars erupt into an initial cusp-to-cusp relationship. This may be rectified by early closure of the lower anthropoid space or by later utilisation of the leeway space.

There are two recognised mechanisms whereby this transient abnormality may be corrected spontaneously. The so-called 'early mechanism' involves mesial drift of the lower first and second deciduous molars into the lower anthropoid space under the driving force of the erupting permanent molar which can then take up a normal relationship with the upper (Fig. 2.4). Similar mesial drift does not occur in the upper arch because the anthropoid space is mesial to the canine which is usually locked by the occlusion.

The second, or 'late mechanism' is dependent on the greater discrepancy between the mesio-distal breadths of the lower deciduous molars and the succeeding premolars than is the case in the upper.[16] In both upper and lower jaws, the sum of the mesio-distal breadths of the permanent canines and premolars is almost invariably smaller than the corresponding measurement of the deciduous canines and deciduous molars. This discrepancy is called the 'leeway space'. The average leeway space is 1.7mm on each side in the lower jaw and 0.9mm on each side in the upper although great variations exist. This greater leeway space in the lower arch may allow the lower first permanent molar to drift mesially to a greater extent than the upper and thus assume a normal inter-digitation when the deciduous molars are shed (see Fig. 2.4).

When the permanent incisors first erupt at about 7 years, a transitional open bite may persist for some months as the teeth erupt and come under the influence of the lips, tongue and cheeks.[17] This open bite will close without treatment (Fig. 2.5).

In the majority of children, the permanent incisor teeth erupt in crowded positions. The combined mesio-distal breadths of the permanent incisors exceeds their deciduous predecessors by about 7mm in the upper jaw and 5mm in the lower jaw.[5] In the upper arch, the lateral incisors generally develop on the palatal side of the centrals and deciduous canines. In the lower arch, the lateral incisors may also erupt lingual to the line of the arch and there is a tendency for the lower incisors to assume a zigzag relationship in the form of the letter M or W. Lower incisors almost invariably procline as they erupt and make some space for themselves in this way.[18,19] Anthropoid and other spaces between the deciduous incisors contribute to the accommodation of the larger permanent teeth. The fact that permanent incisors are generally more proclined and thicker labio-lingually than their deciduous predecessors, means that they occupy an arc of a larger circle which also gives space for their alignment. This is particularly relevant in the upper arch.[5] Some additional space is also forthcoming from lateral jaw growth which seems to occur just before or at the time of eruption of the permanent incisors and may be associated with spacing between the roots of the deciduous teeth.

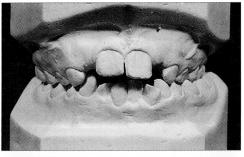

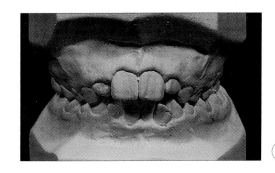

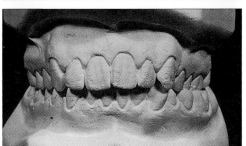

Fig. 2.5 Spontaneous closure of transitional open bite. (a) age 7 years (b) age 8 years (c) age 12 years.

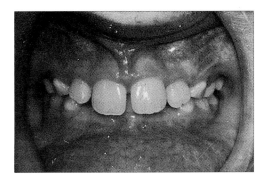

Fig. 2.6 The 'ugly duckling' stage.

The gradual increase in spaces between the crowns of deciduous incisors which might be expected to result from jaw growth between the ages of 2.5 and 6 years does not seem to occur. According to Baume,[20] arches which are spaced at 2.5 years will show the same spaces at 5.5 years and arches which have no spaces at age 2.5 years will not develop spaces during this period.

Another transient abnormality which frequently troubles parents is a mid-line diastema between the permanent central incisors when they first erupt. This may close on eruption of the lateral incisors or may be associated with the lateral fanning of the upper incisors called the 'ugly duckling stage' (Fig. 2.6). It is said to be due to the developing permanent canine teeth being closely applied to the upper part of the lateral incisor roots which results in a distal inclination of the crowns. As the name suggests, spontaneous correction is the rule in these cases. Further eruption of the canine teeth produces pressure on the distal aspect of the lateral incisor crowns which become more upright and any mid-line diastema which still exists tends to close.[21] When the midline diastema is large and persistent, however, radiography to exclude the presence of a supernumerary tooth between the roots of the central incisors is a wise precaution.

Between the ages of 10 and 12 years, with eruption of the premolar and canine teeth, there is a race for space. The first molars are already established at the back of the mouth and the incisors at the front. It is usually a case of first come, first served, so that the early-erupting premolars in the upper arch often leave the canine crowded out in cases where there is primary crowding (a disproportion between the size of teeth, size of jaw and arch perimeter). In the lower arch, however, crowding of the late-erupting second premolar is a consequence of premature loss of the second deciduous molar (secondary crowding) because the second deciduous molar is almost invariably larger than the second premolar and normally maintains space for its permanent successor. Lower second premolars which do become crowded have an amazing capacity for forcing their way into the mouth providing they are in the line of the arch.

Many premolars are rotated when they first appear in the mouth but there is a tendency for many of these rotations to be corrected spontaneously as further eruption occurs.[22]

Functional permanent dentition
Good occlusion at age 18 is shown in Fig. 2.7

Following the attainment of occlusion, teeth continue to erupt and tend to drift in a mesial direction. Between the ages of 13 and 18 years there is an average increase in lower arch crowding and forward movement of lower first molars.[23] There is a correlation between this mesial movement, the development of incisor crowding and diminution of molar crowding in the postadolescent period. The continued forward growth of the mandible after cessation of maxillary growth may lead to retroclination and crowding of lower incisors if they are restrained by the upper incisors when the overbite is substantial.[24] Extremes of mandibular rotation in a backward or forward direction during growth have also been implicated in postadolescent crowding of lower incisors[25] together with other factors such as interproximal periodontal tension,[26] the anterior component of force[27] and increasing lip pressure.[28,29] The role of eruption or attempted eruption of third molars in the development of incisor crowding is unclear, but the presence of a third molar seems to be associated with a tendency to crowding in the same quadrant.[30,31]

Improvements and disimprovements in occlusal development

Features of occlusal development which tend to improve or are of little consequence:

- Post-normal relationship of the gum pads at birth;
- Unusual order of eruption;
- Unusual timing of eruption, within limits;
- Spaced deciduous incisors;
- Slight post-normality of first permanent molars on eruption;
- The ugly duckling stage of development;
- Transitional open bite ;
- Increased overbite when deciduous and permanent incisors first erupt;
- Premolar rotations.

Features of occlusal development which tend to deteriorate:

- Crowded incisors after eruption of premolars and second molars.

The aetiology of malocclusion

The aetiology of malocclusion may be considered under the headings shown in Fig. 2.8. The skeletal pattern or relationship of the jaw bases is largely under genetic control, and it has long been an article of orthodontic dogma that this relationship may not be influenced by orthodontic appliances. On the other hand, there is growing evidence that the facial morphology may be moulded to an uncertain extent by posture, function and functional appliances, or by heavy forces applied through extra-oral traction.[32–34] This question is addressed in Chapter 4.

Much the same sort of debate rages over the possibility of modifying the influence of the soft tissues (the lips, tongue and cheeks) on the dentition and is discussed in Chapter 5.

It is, however, in the realms of crowding and malocclusions associated with local factors (Fig. 2.9) that interceptive orthodontics can be practised most fruitfully. Space maintenance, increasing the arch perimeter, or extraction of teeth can solve or minimise crowding problems. Something can be done about missing teeth, supernumerary teeth, premature loss of deciduous teeth and loss of permanent teeth. Interceptive techniques can influence developing impactions, diastemata associated with abnormal fraena, malocclusions due to habits and local pathological conditions which affect the alignment or relationship of the teeth.

In this age of prevention, most dentists encourage good dietary habits and practise local and general caries prevention. No less important is examination of the patient for the early signs of malocclusion. If incipient malocclusion is to be seen it must first be sought.

Although the interceptive orthodontist must be ever-vigilant, there are particular times when he can identify developing malocclusions most readily. The first is shortly after completion of the deciduous dentition at 3 years, the second is at about 7–9 years when the

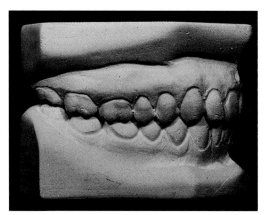

Fig. 2.7 Good occlusion at age 18 years. Same patient as Figs 2.2 and 2.3.

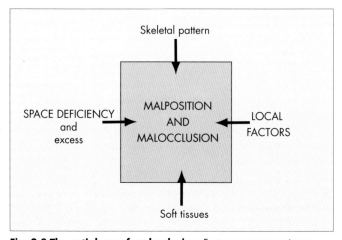

Fig. 2.8 The aetiology of malocclusion. Factors most responsive to interception are in capital letters.

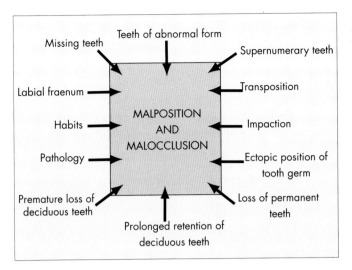

Fig. 2.9 Local factors in the aetiology of malocclusion.

first permanent molars will normally have erupted and the permanent incisors should be erupting, and the third is at about 11–12 years when the premolars, second molars and canines should be coming into the oral cavity.

The fact that these ages of special vigilance do exist has led to the proposal, which is discussed in Chapter 10 and implemented in Chapter 11, that the child population should be screened at these ages and interceptive measures applied where appropriate. While shortage of manpower and finance may delay the introduction of this measure on a community basis, there is no reason why the general dental practitioner should not start screening his patients today if he does not already do so.

References

1 Clinch L. Variation in the degree of overbite between birth and three years. *Dent Record* 1938; **58**: 585–597.

2 Leighton B C. The early development of normal occlusion. *Eur Ortho Soc Trans* 1975: 67–77.

3 Thilander B, Rönning O. *Introduction to orthodontics.* Stockholm: Tandläkarförlaget 1985.

4 Leighton B C. The value of prophecy in orthodontics. *Trans Br Soc Study Orthod* 1971: 1–14.

5 Moorees CFA. *The dentition of the growing child.* Cambridge, Massachusetts: Harvard University Press; 1959.

6 Leighton B C. The early signs of malocclusion. *Eur Orthod Soc Trans* 1969: 353–368.

7 Friel S. The development of ideal occlusion of the gum pads and the teeth. *Am J Orthod* 1954; **40**: 196–227.

8 Clinch L. An analysis of serial models between three and eight years of age. *Dent Record* 1951; **71**: 61–72.

9 Bonnar E M E. Aspects of the transition from deciduous to permanent dentitions. *Dental Practit* 1956; **7**: 42–54.

10 Hurme VO. Ranges of normalcy in the eruption of permanent teeth. *J Dent Children* 1949; **16**: 11–15.

11 Knott VB and Meridith HV. Statistics on eruption of the permanent dentition from serial data for North American white children. *Angle Orthod* 1966; **36**: 68–79.

12 Garn SM, Sandusky ST, Nagy JM, Trowbridge FL. Negro-Caucasoid differences in permanent tooth emergence at a constant income level. *Arch Oral Biol* 1973; **18**: 609–615.

13 Lavelle CLB. The timing of tooth emergence in four population samples - a cross-sectional study. *J Dent* 1976; **4**: 231–236.

14 Virtanen JI, Bloigu RS, Larmas MA. Timing of eruption of permanent teeth: standard Finnish documents. *Community Dent Oral Epidemiol* 1994; **22**: 286–288.

15 Kochhar R, Richardson A. The chronology and sequence of eruption of human permanent teeth in Northern Ireland. *Int J Paed Dent* 1998; **8**: 243–252.

16 Nance HN. Limitations of orthodontic treatment. 1. Mixed dentition diagnosis and treatment. *Am J Orthod Oral Surg* 1947; **33**: 177–223 and 255–301.

17 Richardson A. A classification of open bites. *Eur J Orthod* 1981; **3**: 289–296.

18 Adams CP, Richardson A. An assessment of the relationship of the pre- and post-eruptive lower incisor position to the facial pattern by serial cephalometric radiography. *Eur Orthod Soc Trans* 1967: 213–223.

19 McMullan RE, Richardson A. Eruptive changes in the axial inclination of lower incisor teeth – a longitudinal study. *J Irish Dent Assoc* 1990; **36**: 289–296.

20 Baume L I. Physiological tooth migration and its significance for the development of occlusion. *J Dent Res* 1950; **29**: 123–132.

21 Broadbent B H. Ontogenic development of occlusion. *Angle Orthod* 1941; **11**: 223–241.

22 McMullan RE, Richardson A. Spontaneous changes in rotation of premolar teeth from eruption until the established dentition. *Eur J Orthod* 1991; **13**: 392–396.

23 Richardson, ME. Late lower arch crowding: facial growth or forward drift? *Eur J Orthod* 1979; **1**: 219–225.

24 Björk A, Palling M. Adolescent growth changes in sagittal jaw relation, alveolar prognathy and incisal inclination. *Acta odontol Scand* 1954; **12**: 201–232.

25 Björk A. Prediction of mandibular growth rotation. *Am J Orthod* 1969; **55**: 585–599

26 Southard TE, Southard KA, Tolley EA. Periodontal forces: a potential cause of relapse. *Am J Orthod Dentofac Orthop* 1992; **101**: 221–227.

27 Southard TE, Behrents RG, Tolley EA. The anterior component of occlusal force. Part 2. Relationship with dental malalignment. *Am J Orthod Dentofac Orthop* 1990; **97**: 41–44.

28 Vig PS, Cohen AM. Vertical growth of the lips: a serial cephalometric study. *Am J Orthod* 1979; **75**: 405–415.

29 Subtelny JD, Sakuda M. Muscle function, oral malformation, and growth changes. *Am J Orthod* 1966; **52**: 495–517.

30 Richardson ME. The role of the third molar in the cause of late lower crowding: A review. *Am J Orthod Dentofac Orthop* 1989; **95**: 79–83.

31 Vego L. A longitudinal study of mandibular arch perimeter. *Angle Orthod* 1962; **32**: 187–192.

32 Forsberg C-M, Odenrick L. Skeletal and soft tissue response to activator treatment. *Eur J Orthod* 1981; **3**: 247–253.

33 Mills J R E. The effect of orthodontic treatment on the skeletal pattern. *Br J Orthod* 1978; **5**: 133–143.

34 Fränkel R A. A functional approach to orofacial orthopaedics. *Br J Orthod* 1980; **7**: 41–51.

35 Foster TD, Grundy MC, Lavelle CLB. Changes in occlusion in the primary dentition between 2fi and 5fi years of age. *Euro Ortho Soc Trans* 1972: 75–84.

36 Savara BS, Steen JC. Timing and sequence of eruption of permanent teeth in a longitudinal sample of children from Oregon. *J Amer Dent Assoc* 1978; **97**: 209–214.

37 Sillman JH. Dimensional changes of the dental arches; longitudinal study from birth to 25 years. *Am J Orthod* 1964; **50**: 824–842.

Summary of evidence for Chapter 2

Topic	Findings	Author/s
Overbite	Vertical space between gum pads allows normal dental overbite. Absence of the space unfavourable for mandibular growth.	Clinch 1938.[1] Longitudinal study of 25 children from birth to 3yrs.
Occlusal changes	Overbite and overjet at birth are poor predictors of future arch relationship. Deep overbite in mature deciduous dentition closely correlated with permanent overbite.	Leighton 1971.[4] Longitudinal cast and cephalometric study of 529 British children from birth to 16yrs.
Changes in crowding & occlusion	Average decrease in arch length (from incisors to second deciduous molars). Mean circumference increases in upper, decreases in lower. Average changes in space conditions are 'useful abstractions at best' Stresses individual variations and the value of longitudinal supervision.	Moorees 1959.[5] Longitudinal cast studies of 2 series: 132 from birth to 18 yrs and 52 from 5 to 18yrs.
Occlusal changes	Unilateral crossbites often improve, bilateral crossbites rarely do. **Deciduous spaces** **Permanent crowding** 0 — 2 in 3 chance < 3mm — 1 in 2 chance 3–6mm — 1 in 5 chance > 6mm — Little chance	Leighton 1969.[6] Longitudinal model study of 57F,46M between 5.5 and 13.5yrs.
Occlusion ideals and maturation	Space for larger permanent incisors made by increased arch breadth, root spacing of deciduous incisors, labial inclination of permanent incisors. Forward movement of lower deciduous molars relative to upper contributes to development of ideal permanent molar occlusion.	Friel 1954.[7] Classical description of occlusal development based on Clinch[1] material, 214 chimpanzee skulls and radiographs of 369 children between 3 and 5 yrs.
Occlusal changes	Normal molar occlusion may be attained at completion of deciduous dentition, before or during eruption of 6s, or during eruption of incisors. Sides behave independently.	Bonnar 1956.[9] 6-monthly casts of 58 children from shedding of first incisor to full eruption of permanent incisors.
Eruption ages	Derived standards for white children living in temperate zone. Females before males. No sex difference in variability of eruption age. Limited by lack of data in some papers.	Hurme 1949.[10] Meta-analysis of 24 papers totalling 93,000 children from Europe and North America.
Eruption ages and sequences	Most common sequences Upper: 6,1,2,4,3,5,7 and 6,1,2,4,5,3,7 Lower: 1,6,2,4,3,5,7, and 1,6,2,3,4,5,7	Knott & Meridith 1966.[11] Longitudinal study of 107 children in Iowa.
Eruption ages	Negroes before Caucasians. Racial differences exceed socio-economic.	Garn et al 1973.[12] Cross-sectional study of 3,868 American Negro and 5,788 American Caucasians.
Eruption ages	Variation in age of eruption greatest for upper lateral in males, upper first premolar in females.	Lavelle 1976.[13] Cross-sectional study of 4,000 children in 4 English areas.
Eruption ages	Little difference between contralateral teeth. Females before males. Lower before upper. Later eruption in high fluoride areas.	Virtanen et al 1994.[14] Cross-sectional study of 911 children in Finland.
Eruption ages and sequences	Results quoted refer to cases without premature loss. Females before males except for second molars. Lower before upper except for premolars. No difference between sides. Premature loss of deciduous teeth delays age of eruption except upper premolars. Most common sequence of eruption unique to the subject.	Kochhar & Richardson 1998.[15] Longitudinal study of 276 children in Northern Ireland.
Lower incisor inclinations	Lower incisors were always more proclined after eruption than before. The average difference was 13°.	Adams & Richardson 1967.[18] Longitudinal cephalometric study of 24F,26M between 5 and 11yrs.

Topic (continued)	Findings	Author/s
Lower incisor inclinations	Greatest rate of proclination in first year after eruption. Diminution in proclination not related to occlusal contact.	McMullan & Richardson 1990.[19] Longitudinal cephalometric study of 18F,14M from 5 to10 yrs.
Occlusal changes	Primate spaces present. No change in spacing between deciduous teeth or deciduous arch dimensions after 3yrs. Terminal planes remained constant.	Baume 1950.[20] Longitudinal cast study of 30 from 3 to 5.5yrs.
Dental and facial growth related	Mid-sagittal points grow in straight lines except nasion. Malocclusions are caused by deficient facial growth which may catch up after illness. Ugly duckling described. Resolution is due to lateral development of apical base. 'Bimaxillary dental protrusion' is really due to retruded facial skeleton.	Broadbent 1941.[21] Descriptive paper. Longitudinal cephalometric study of 5,000 Cleveland children from birth to adulthood. Bolton/Brush Foundations.
Lower arch crowding	Increasing crowding related to forward movement of first molars. Lower incisors proclined.	Richardson ME 1979.[23] Longitudinal study of 51 children with third molars at ages 13 and 18yrs.
Lower arch crowding	Increasing mandibular prognathism relative to maxilla during growth. Lower incisors retroclined.	Björk & Palling 1954.[24] Longitudinal study of 243 males between 12 and 20yrs.
Lower arch crowding	Crowding related to extremes of clockwise and counterclockwise mandibular growth rotation.	Björk 1969.[25] Longitudinal study of 243 males between 12 and 20yrs.
Periodontal forces	Continuous periodontal force compressing proximal contacts. Force increased under occlusal load.	Southard et al 1992.[26] Tension transducer measurements of 10 subjects.
Periodontal forces	Significant correlation between interproximal force and mandibular anterior crowding.	Southard et al 1990.[27] Tension transducer measurements of 15 subjects.
Lip growth	Lips grow up to 19yrs. Lip growth exceeds growth in anterior facial height.	Vig & Cohen 1979.[28] Longitudinal cephalometric study of 50 subjects between 4 and 20yrs.
Lower arch crowding	Presence of third molars related to greater crowding.	Vego 1962.[31] Longitudinal study of 40 with and 25 without third molars between 12 and 17yrs.
Functional appliances (Andresen)	Significant decrease in SNA, ANB, and overjet in treated cases. Good lip balance after treatment except in pre-existing extremes of mandibular angle and poor chin/lip and nose relationship.	Forsberg & Odenrick 1981.[32] Longitudinal study of 47 cases with 31 controls.
Functional appliances	0.5–1.0mm additional mandibular growth on average.	Mills 1978.[33] Review.
Occlusal changes	Mean reduction in overjet and overbite but wide individual variations. 66% of molar relationships unchanged, 24% relative mesial movement of lower, 10% relative distal movement of lower.	Foster et al 1972.[35] Longitudinal study of 70 British subjects at ages 2.5 and 5yrs.
Eruption ages and sequences	Most likely sequences Upper: 6,1,2,4,5,3,7 in males 6,1,2,4,3,5,7 in females Lower: 1,6,2,3,4,5,7 in both sexes. Occurred in only 11–13% of subjects	Savara & Steen 1978.[36] Longitudinal study of 287 Caucasian children in Oregon.
Arch dimension changes	Arch length: continuous increase to 25yrs. in males. No change after 14yrs in females. Canine and molar width: continuous increase to 12yrs and 14yrs respectively .	Sillman 1964.[37] Longitudinal study of 65 children from birth to 25yrs.

Radiography and radiographic interpretation

Radiographic assessment is important in the practice of interceptive orthodontics.

At the simplest level, radiographs will reveal the presence and positions of unerupted teeth of the normal series and give essential information about the presence of any supernumerary elements or pathology. More specifically, radiographs will reveal deficiencies of calcification such as enamel hypoplasia, dental caries, the extent and approximal shape of restorations, and abnormalities of the roots of teeth such as dilacerations, incomplete apices, resorption, ankylosis and apical pathology.

Beyond that, cephalometric radiographs can give additional information on facial morphology, the relationship of the jaw bases to one another and the relationship of the dentition to the face.

The risks and benefits of radiography must be taken into account. Of the total radiation received by the British population, 87% is from natural sources and 12% from the use of radiation in medicine. Radiation in dentistry constitutes a small fraction of the total medical figure. Although the relative risks from dental radiography seem small, radiographic examination should never become routine and, in any event, it has been shown that routine radiographic screening as compared with clinical examination with selective radiography has little effect on treatment plans for children aged 11–12 years.[1]

Guidelines for the use of radiographs in orthodontics are neatly summarised in a publication from the British Orthodontic Society.[2] Another useful document giving the do's and don'ts for good radiological practice is distributed by the Faculty of GDPs (UK).[3]

From the diagnostic standpoint, radiographs provide important information following clinical detection of abnormalities and may allow informed interceptive treatment of many of these. Teeth which have not appeared in the mouth on time, persistent midline diastema, retained deciduous molars and unerupted unpalpable maxillary canines are obvious examples. Similarly, many interceptive treatments involve timely extraction of teeth and depend on the presence of sound unerupted teeth in favourable positions which can only be demonstrated radiographically.

All of the many radiographic views have advantages and shortcomings which are listed below. In pragmatic terms, practitioners are likely to be limited in their choice by the power of the available x-ray generator and in some cases by the preference of the surgeon with whom they work.

Intra-oral radiographs

Intra-oral or periapical films measuring 31×41mm or 22×35mm are difficult to accommodate in a small mouth and often only the crowns of unerupted teeth are shown. Since eight to ten films are needed to cover the dentition of a child, intra-oral films have limited and localised value in orthodontics. The exposures are made with a standard dental tube working at 60–70KVp. A diligent member of staff should mount these views correctly on a transparent sheet or in commercially available frames. Otherwise these sets of films are like an irritating shower of confetti in the patient's notes and must be sorted each time they are used, giving an opportunity for error. The blip on the film is towards the tube. Some films have no blip but the figures in one corner assist orientation.

Providing the film is closely applied to the object radiographed without bending or is used with modern film holders, good intra-oral films can give excellent detail with little distortion (Fig. 3.1).[4]

Bitewing radiographs are taken on films measuring 31×41mm for adults or 22×35mm for children. As the name implies, the patient bites on a tab or film packet holder which retains the film parallel with the line of the arch in close proximity to the lingual sides of the teeth. The tube is angulated downwards between 5 and 8 degrees and at right angles to the film in the horizontal plane. Both upper and lower teeth are shown on the film, without superimposition of the contact areas. Bitewing films are used for detection of approximal decay or faulty restorations and can be used to demonstrate interproximal bone levels (Fig. 3.2)

Anterior occlusal radiographs

The upper or lower standard or anterior occlusal view is taken on film measuring 57×76mm. The film is placed between the upper and lower teeth and the tube placed on the bridge of the nose and angulated downwards 65–70 degrees to the film for the upper view. For the lower, the tube is placed on the point of the chin and angulated upwards 45 degrees to the film. Exposures can be made with the standard dental set. These views show pictures of upper or lower incisors and canines (which are frequently elongated) in convenient form. The blip on the film is towards the tube. Some surgeons like this view (Fig. 3.3).

Vertex occlusal radiographs

The Vertex occlusal view is taken with the tube placed about 1.5" behind the hair-line and angulated downwards along the long axes of the upper incisor teeth. Films 57×76mm are contained in cassettes with intensifying screens to enhance the radiographic exposure. The cassettes are enveloped in cellophane or plastic bags for reasons of hygiene. The cassette is held between the teeth at 90 degrees to the teeth of special interest. The object is to produce a plan view of the upper arch with the frontal bone thrown forward so that it is not superimposed over the upper incisors. Exposures can be made

with the standard intra-oral x-ray set. The left or right side should be marked. The high exposure and the orientation of the beam towards the eyes, thyroid gland and reproductive organs has made this view unpopular. The radiograph gives a rather indistinct picture of the teeth in cross section (Fig. 3.4).

Lateral jaw radiographs

Oblique lateral jaw views are taken on films measuring 13×18cm contained in a cassette with intensifying screens. They can give an adequate but enlarged view of the teeth posterior to and including the canine. Positioning of the patient may be facilitated with a hinged board.[5] By alternately covering half of the film with a lead sheet it is possible to show both sides of the mouth conveniently on one piece of film. These are sometimes called bimolar views (Fig. 3.5). Care must be taken to label the sides. Exposures can be made using a standard dental set but any 'clip on' rectangular collumator should be removed.

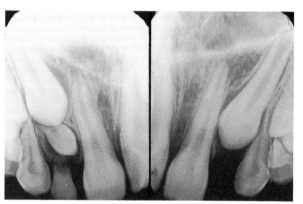

Fig. 3.1 Intra-oral radiographs. The upper left permanent lateral incisor is absent. There is a diminutive permanent lateral incisor on the right side with retention of the corresponding deciduous tooth. Both permanent canines are developing in mesial positions.

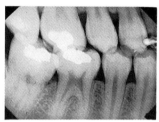

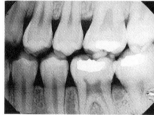

Fig 3.2 Bitewing radiographs.

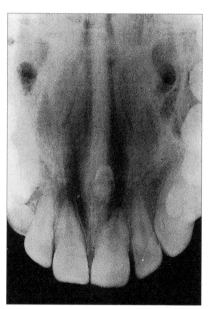

Fig. 3.3 Upper standard or anterior occlusal radiograph. There is an unerupted inverted mesiodens.

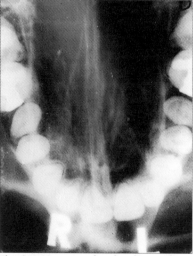

Fig. 3.4 Vertex occlusal radiograph.

Fig. 3.5 Oblique lateral views. Both lower second premolars are hypoplastic and distally inclined especially on the left side where the first molar has been extracted. All four third molars are unerupted as are the maxillary canines, all the lower premolars and the upper left second premolar.

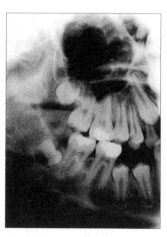

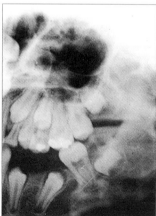

Panoramic tomographs

Panoramic tomographs (Orthopan, OPT) are very useful in interceptive orthodontics but need a dedicated generator and special equipment which, in some cases, is combined with a cephalostat. Tube and patient positioning is standardised. The effective dose of radiation is approximately equivalent to four or five peri-apical radiographs. The sides must be marked. These views are easy to take and give a general but distorted and magnified view of the dentition in convenient form (Fig. 3.6). Artefacts are frequent. Ghost images from the other side of the mouth and cervical spine are superimposed over the structures in focus. Air shadows may simulate caries. The pictures are more reliable towards the back of the mouth than at the front where the shallow tomographic depth (image layer, focal trough, focal corridor) and super-imposition of the cervical spine may make interpretation difficult.

The representation of crowding or spacing and the occlusion on an orthopan (OPT) film is very unreliable, the latter because the mandible is usually protruded in taking the film. Some authorities, however, argue that tomograms for orthodontic purposes should be taken with the teeth in occlusion since the benefits of correct occlusal registration outweigh any loss of detail in the incisal region.[6] Some machines (split-mode Panorex) show two views of the incisor region which can be used in the method of parallax. Orthopantomographs showing development of the dentition between the ages of 4 and 16 years are shown in Figures 3.7–3.15.

Cephalometric radiographs

Cephalometric radiography needs a high output tube working at 90 or 100KVp which can be combined with an orthopantomogram. The relationship of the tube, the head and the film holder is standardised. Cephalometric views are taken with the tube five feet from the patient in order to reduce the degree of enlargement. The general order of enlargement on the lateral view is about 8% for a structure in the mid-sagittal plane. Films 10"×12" or 18×24 cm are contained in cassettes with intensifying screens. Many cephalostats incorporate a grid, pre-focused at 5 feet, to filter out secondary radiation which can fog the film. There is usually an aluminium wedge which is adjusted to cover the projection of the nose, chin and lips so that these soft tissues will show on the film with an exposure appropriate for calcified tissue. The lateral view, showing the patient in profile, is the most popular, but most cephalostats can be adjusted for a standardised postero-anterior view and some can be used to take reproducible views at any given rotation. Most cephalometric exposures are made with the teeth in occlusion (Fig. 3.16)

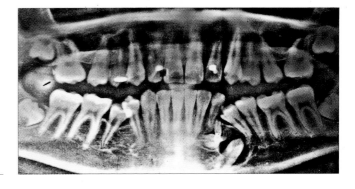

Fig. 3.6 Panoramic tomograph. The lower left permanent canine is unerupted and has a dentigerous follicular cyst round its crown. The corresponding deciduous tooth is retained with two supernumerary teeth near the apex. Both upper first permanent molars are missing. All four third molars are present. Some teeth have restorations.

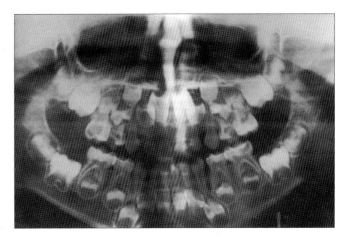

Fig. 3.7 Orthopantomograph (OPT) showing dental development in a Caucasian male between his fourth and fifth birthdays. All deciduous teeth have erupted. Some are carious. The crowns of the first permanent molars have calcified and root formation has started. The crowns of the lower incisors are almost completely formed and calcification has commenced in the crowns of the other teeth.

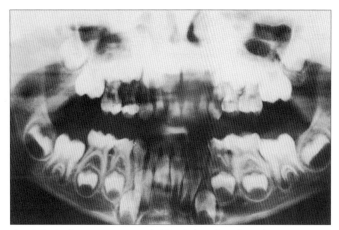

Fig. 3.8 Orthopantomograph (OPT) showing dental development in a Caucasian male between his fifth and sixth birthdays. Between one third and half of the roots of the first permanent molars have formed, root formation of the lower incisors has started, and the crowns of the permanent upper incisors, canines, premolars and second molars are between one third and half calcified.

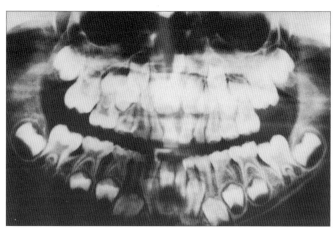

Fig. 3.9 Orthopantomograph (OPT) showing dental development in a Caucasian male between his sixth and seventh birthdays. The first permanent molars and lower central incisors are at various stages of eruption, half of the roots of the first molars have formed and crown formation of canines, premolars and second molars is approaching completion.

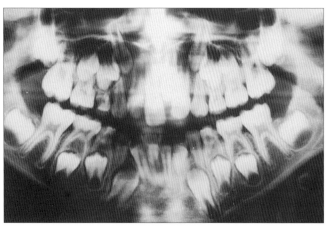

Fig. 3.10 Orthopantomograph (OPT) showing dental development in a Caucasian female between her seventh and eighth birthdays. Eruption of the upper left central incisor is delayed. The first permanent molars and permanent incisors have erupted, more than two thirds of the roots of the lower first molars and between one third and half of the roots of the canines have formed. Crown formation of premolars and second molars is complete.

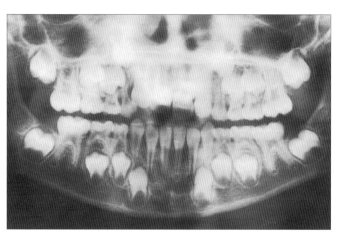

Fig. 3.11 Orthopantomograph (OPT) showing dental development in a Caucasian male between his eighth and ninth birthdays. The first permanent molars and permanent incisors have erupted, the apices of the first permanent molars are still open, crown formation of canines, premolars and second molars is complete and root formation is starting. The crypts of the third molars are visible.

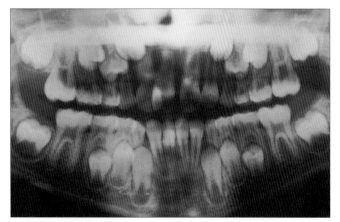

Fig. 3.12 Orthopantomograph (OPT) showing dental development in a Caucasian male between his ninth and tenth birthdays. The first permanent molars and incisors have erupted The apices of the first permanent molars are almost complete, root formation of the lower second molars has started, one third of root formation has been achieved in the premolars and between half and two thirds in the lower canines. Resorption of the deciduous canines and molars teeth has started.

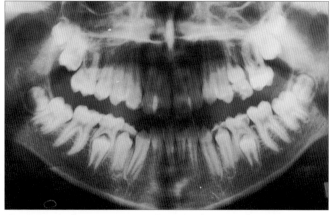

Fig. 3.13 Orthopantomograph (OPT) showing dental development in a Caucasian male close to his eleventh birthday. The first permanent molars, incisors, lower canines, upper first premolars and upper right second premolar have erupted, the upper canines and lower second molars are erupting. Resorption of the remaining deciduous molars is advancing and the related premolars are moving towards the mouth cavity.

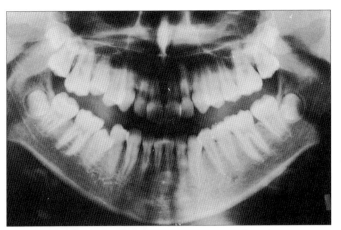

Fig. 3.14 Orthopantomograph (OPT) showing dental development in a Caucasian female between her eleventh and twelfth birthdays. All teeth with the exception of the third molars have erupted, the second premolars and second molars have open apices, and crown formation of the third molars is almost complete. The lower right second premolar is rotated and only partially erupted on account of crowding subsequent to early loss of the lower right second deciduous molar.

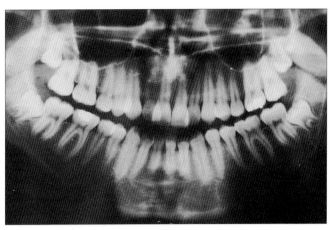

Fig. 3.15 Orthopantomograph (OPT) showing dental development in a Caucasian male at age 16. With the exception of the third molars, all teeth of the permanent series have erupted and have closed apices. The crowns of the third molars are fully calcified and root formation has commenced. There is a supplemental tooth distal to the third molar in the upper left quadrant.

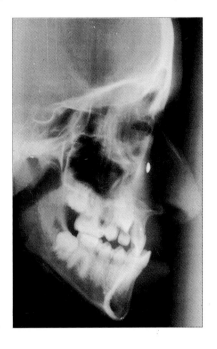

Fig. 3.16 Cephalometric radiograph. There is a Class III relationship of the incisor teeth on a mild Class III skeletal pattern. The second molars and maxillary canines are unerupted.

The advantage of a single lateral cephalometric film is that it shows the teeth, soft tissues and alveolar and basal bones in correct relation to each other (but with the right and left sides superimposed). Within limits, it can be used for accurate measurement of such parameters as the inclinations and relationships of the incisor teeth, the basal bones and the soft tissues. Today, cephalometric films are usually analysed by computer using digitised co-ordinates so that a correction factor for enlargement can be applied easily. Computer analysis is quick and the accuracy of the digitiser far exceeds the ability of the human eye to identify most cephalometric points.[7] Most cephalometric programs will predict the face after orthodontic or surgical treatment, presuming that the movement of the lips and cheeks will correspond exactly with the dental and skeletal changes induced by the treatment. Since cephalometric views are standardised, a pair of films taken on different occasions may be compared and the changes during growth, treatment or relapse can be measured.

Cephalometric films are the most commonly used research tool in orthodontics. Following clinical examination, most orthodontists would see an orthopantomograph and a cephalometric film as a basic set of radiographs for orthodontic diagnosis. Few dentists have a cephalostat and most will have to rely on clinical estimation of the shape of the face and inclinations of incisor teeth. An orthopantomogram is more common in practice and is a very useful and convenient tool for anyone who practices orthodontics, interceptive or otherwise. However, most of the information in an orthopantomograph can be seen on bimolar views supplemented by anterior occlusal or intra-oral views, all of which can be taken using a standard dental tube.

Interpretation of radiographs

Viewing conditions are important. A viewer inclined at about 30 degrees makes for unstrained examination by the seated clinician and easy demonstration to a patient or parent. Ideally, radiographs should be viewed against a north light although this is not essential. Darkening the room and excluding light from the viewer round the radiograph has a significant effect on perception of the image.

Initial examination of radiographs is prompted by the clinical findings but it is useful to have an additional routine for detection of unsuspected anomalies:

- Identify each tooth, note absences and supernumeraries.
- Examine each crown for morphology, degree of calcification, and restorations. Is there invagination or hypoplasia?
- Examine each root for development, morphology, dilaceration, apical pathology and resorption.
- Is the follicular space of unerupted teeth enlarged?
- Compare the stage of dental development with known standards (see Figs 3.7–3.15)
- Is the eruption of any tooth delayed?
- Is resorption of the roots of deciduous teeth proceeding normally?
- Examine the inclination of each tooth and its relationship to adjoining teeth. Is there impaction?
- Are the bone levels normal?
- Is the interpremaxillary suture particularly prominent?
- A last look for pathology.

Radiographs are two dimensional shadows of three dimensional objects and it may be difficult to locate teeth in the bucco-lingual plane of space. Three dimensional localisation is frequently needed for unerupted second premolars, maxillary canines and supernumerary teeth. While clinical experience and palpation shows that the majority of these are on the palatal or lingual side of the arch, there are radiographic methods of locating them more precisely as follows:

- A pair of radiographic views at precisely or approximately right angles to each other, such as lateral and posterio-anterior cephalometric films, an orthopantomograph and vertex occlusal, a lateral jaw and vertex occlusal or an intra-oral and vertex occlusal. The cephalometric pair has the advantage that the views are precisely at right angles to each other so that the length of an unerupted tooth can be calculated using solid geometry.[8] The disadvantage is that unerupted teeth are superimposed on other structures and special equipment in the form of a cephalostat is required. Most of the other pairs of films can be taken with a dental set but all include the vertex-occlusal view which is hazardous on account of the high radiation and angulation of the beam.
- Two views taken at different angles (the tube shift or parallax method) are most commonly used for unerupted maxillary canines. Traditionally this is done by placing an intra-oral film on the palatal side of the unerupted tooth and making an exposure with the x-ray beam directed distally, then placing a second film in the same place and making an exposure with the x-ray beam directed mesially. The principle of the method can be demonstrated by holding up the forefinger of each hand, one behind the other and moving the head from side to side. The more distant finger appears to move in the same direction as the head relative to the other finger. The two radiographs are interpreted by comparing the movement of the unerupted canine relative to the first premolar or lateral incisor. If the unerupted canine appears to move in the same direction as the tube, it is palatally placed (Fig. 3.17).

Many patients will have a pantomograph for other reasons. This film can be paired with an anterior occlusal view for the method of parallax in the vertical plane. The tube shift in this pair is from 8 degrees upward in the pantomograph to a higher position and 65–70 degree downward inclination for the anterior occlusal view. If the vertical movement of the unerupted canine relative to the incisor teeth is in the same direction as the tube, the canine is palatally placed (Fig. 3.18).

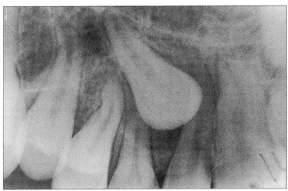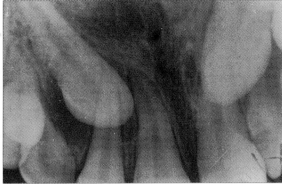

Fig. 3.17 The method of parallax. As the tube is moved distally from the right view to the left, the upper right canine seems to move, relative to the lateral incisor, in the same direction as the tube. The upper right canine is on the palatal side of the lateral incisor.

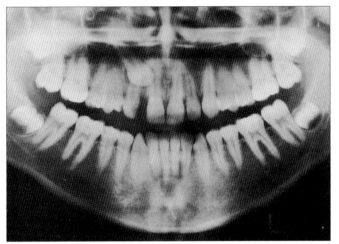

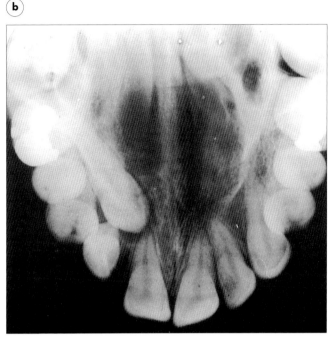

Fig. 3.18 Parallax in the vertical plane. As the tube position changes from low in the orthopantomograph (a) to high in the anterior occlusal view (b) the unerupted upper right canine seems to move in the same direction relative to the root of the central incisor. The upper right canine is on the palatal side of the central incisor.

References

1 Hintze H, Wenzel A, Williams S. Diagnostic value of clinical examination for the identification of children in need of orthodontic treatment compared with clinical examination and screening pantomography. *Eur J Orthod* 1990; 12: 385–388.

2 Isaacson KG, Jones ML. *Orthodontic radiography: guidelines.* British Orthodontic Society, London: 1994.

3 Selection Criteria for Dental Radiography. Faculty of GDPs (UK), London: 1998.

4 Whiates E, Brown J. An update on dental imaging. *Br Dent J* 1998; 185: 166–172.

5 Adams CP. The oblique lateral jaw radiograph. *Br J Orthod* 1974; 1: 139–142.

6 Fischer-Brandies H. Remarks on the diagnostic advantages of panoramic tomograms obtained with the teeth in occlusion. *Electromedica* 1985; 53: 154–157.

7 Richardson A. A comparison of traditional and computerized methods of cephalometric analysis. *Eur J Orthod* 1981; 3:15–20.

8 Richardson A, McKay C. The unerupted maxillary canine, its clinical level after surgical repositioning. *Br Dent J* 1965; 118: 123–236.

Skeletal relationships, facial growth and growth prediction

The evidence-based findings are summarised on pages 30 and 31.

Skeletal relationships

The teeth and alveolar processes are attached to the basal bones of the maxilla and mandible and the occlusion of the teeth is greatly influenced by the relationship of the basal bones in all three planes of space.

The antero-posterior relationship of the jaw bases is variously called the dental base relationship or skeletal pattern or incisor apical base relationship. Although these terms may not be strictly synonymous, the name 'skeletal pattern' will be used for simplicity to cover all of these. The skeletal pattern may be:

- Class I, where the antero-posterior relationship of mandible to maxilla is normal or ideal.
- Class II, where the mandible is posteriorly placed in relation to the maxilla.
- Class III, where the mandible is anteriorly placed in relation to the maxilla.

These classes are shown in Figures 4.1, 4.2, and 4.3.

The term 'skeletal relationships' takes into account all three planes of space.

Cephalometric analysis

A simple cephalometric analysis is shown in Figure 4.4

Normal cephalometric values and standard deviations for young adult Caucasians having good occlusions are given in Table 4.1

The skeletal pattern is usually quantified by the angle subtended by the anterior limits of the maxilla and mandible (the A and B points respectively) to the sella-nasion line at nasion. Positive values are with A anterior to B. The vertical relationship is measured by the angle between the maxillary and mandibular planes or the percentage contribution of the lower face height (ANS-Me) to the total face height (N-Me) measured vertically. The lateral relationship is rarely measured at all.

The effect of the dentition on the profile is another important measurement which is usually given by the distance from the incisal edge of the most prominent lower incisor to a line joining A to pogonion (A-Po). Positive values are with the lower incisal edge anterior to A-Po. The soft tissue profile is most easily measured by the relationship of the lips to the E line (aesthetic line, in America esthetic line) which joins the tip of the nose to the soft tissue chin.

(a)

(b)

(c)

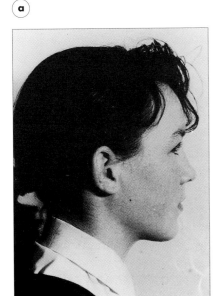
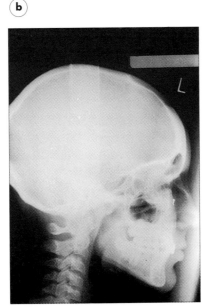
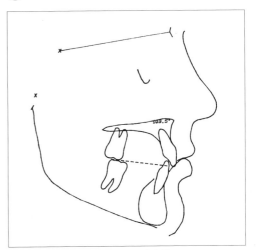

SNA 81.0°   SNB 78.3°   ANB 2.7°
Maxillary/mandibular planes angle 28°
Lower to total facial height 55.1%
Lower incisor to A-Po -0.9 mm.

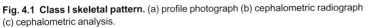

Fig. 4.1 Class I skeletal pattern. (a) profile photograph (b) cephalometric radiograph (c) cephalometric analysis.

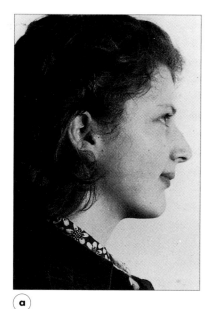
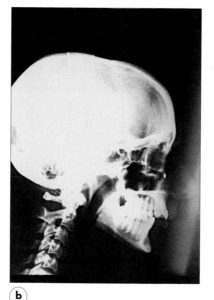
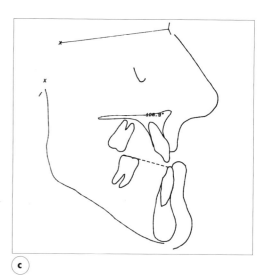

SNA 79.2°   SNB 70.2°   ANB 9.0°
Maxillary/mandibular planes angle 30.5°
Lower to total facial height 55.0%
Lower incisor to A-Po -10.0 mm.

Fig. 4.2 Class II skeletal pattern. (a) profile photograph (b) cephalometric radiograph (c) cephalometric analysis.

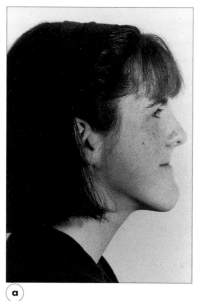
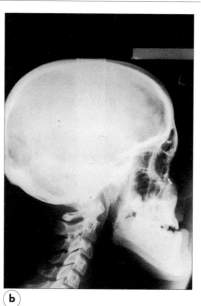

SNA 80.1°   SNB 83.7°   ANB -3.6°
Maxillary/mandibular planes angle 34.0°
Lower to total facial height 64.9%
Lower incisor to A-Po 1.5 mm.

Fig. 4.3 Class III skeletal pattern. (a) profile photograph (b) cephalometric radiograph (c) cephalometric analysis.

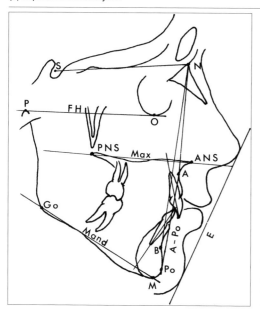

Fig. 4.4 Cephalometric analysis. S, Sella, the centre of the sella turcica. N, Nasion, the junction of the nasal and frontal bones in the midline. O, Orbitale, the lowest point on the outline of the orbit. P, Porion, the highest point on the external auditory meatus. A, the most posterior point on the concave outline of the maxilla labial to the upper incisors. B, the most posterior point on the concave outline of the mandible labial to the lower incisors. Po, the most anterior point on the bony chin. ANS, Anterior nasal spine. PNS, Posterior nasal spine. M, Menton, the lowest point on the bony chin. Go, Gonion, the lowest, most posterior point at the angle of the mandible. Max, Maxillary plane, joining ANS to PNS. Mand, Mandibular plane, joining Go to Me. A–Po, A to pogonion line. E, Aesthetic line, joining the tip of the nose to the most anterior point on the soft tissue chin. FH, the Frankfort horizontal.

Table 4.1 Normal cephalometric values and standard deviations for young adult caucasians having good occlusions. About 2 in 3 of the sample fell within the range +/- one standard deviation of the average.

	Average	Standard deviation
Angle SNA (degrees)	81	3.7
Angle SNB (degrees)	79	3.9
Angle ANB (degrees)	2	1.9
Intermaxillary angle (degrees)	26	5.2
Lower face proportion of total (percent)	55	2.2
Upper incisor inclination (degrees)	110	5.3
Lower incisor inclination (degrees)	89	6.1
Interincisal angle (degrees)	136	9.0
Lower incisor to A-Po (mm)	0	2
Upper lip to E line (mm)	-2	1
Lower lip to E line (mm)	-1	1

Clinical assessment

In the absence of cephalometric facilities, many clinicians successfully rely on clinical judgement of these features.

For the clinical assessment of the skeletal pattern, the patient should be seated upright with the Frankfort plane (the eye-ear plane) horizontal. Very gross skeletal Class II and skeletal Class III patterns can be seen at a glance, as can long or short faces. Smaller antero-posterior discrepancies may be detected by palpating the A and B points with the forefinger and middle finger. (Fig. 4.5) Vertical discrepancies may be estimated by placing the forefinger along the lower border of the mandible and estimating the angle made with the Frankfort plane (the FM angle) (Fig. 4.6).

A more detailed technique is attributed to Ballard.[1] His method depends on three factors:

- The skeletal pattern;
- The inclinations of the upper and lower incisor teeth;
- The overjet.

The argument is that if any two of the above are normal, the third will also be normal. For example, a normal skeletal pattern associated with normally inclined incisors must lead to a normal overjet (the statement is not necessarily true in all circumstances, but it will suffice). Likewise, normally inclined incisors which have a normal overjet must have a normal skeletal pattern.

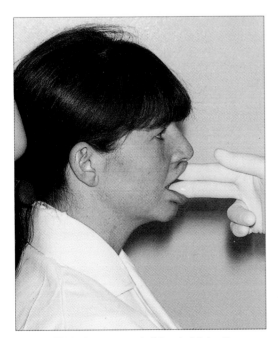

Fig. 4.5 Clinical assessment of the skeletal pattern.

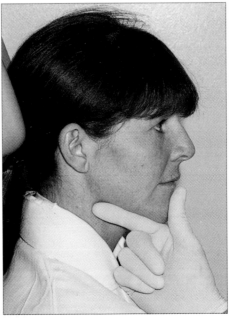

Fig. 4.6 Clinical assessment of the Frankfort-mandibular planes angle (FM angle).

In assessing the skeletal pattern, the inclination of the upper incisors to the Frankfort plane is estimated and mentally adjusted to a normal value (Fig. 4.7). Similarly, the inclination of the lower incisors to the mandibular plane is assessed and mentally adjusted to a normal value (Fig. 4.8). The overjet of these mentally adjusted upper and lower incisors is estimated. If the overjet is normal, the skeletal pattern is normal. If the overjet is increased, the skeletal pattern is Class II. If it is reduced or reversed, the skeletal pattern is Class III.

An important modification concerns the angle between the Frankfort and mandibular planes. If the method is used in a patient with a normal skeletal pattern but an abnormally large FM angle, the lower incisors, mentally adjusted to 90 degrees to the mandibular plane, will lean forward because of the increased FM angle and the patient will be misdiagnosed as having a Class III skeletal pattern. Compensation for variations in the FM angle can be made in the following way : for every degree the FM angle is higher than the normal of 27 degrees, the lower incisors should be mentally adjusted to an angle of 1 degree less than 90 degrees to the mandibular plane. Likewise, for every degree the FM angle is lower than ideal, the lower incisors should be set at an angle of 1 degree more than 90 degrees to the mandibular plane.

With experience, it becomes possible to distinguish mild from gross skeletal discrepancies (Fig. 4.9). The normal overjet is the situation when the mentally adjusted lower incisor is opposite the middle third of the palatal surface of the mentally adjusted upper incisor.

If, following adjustment, the incisal edge of the lower incisor is opposite the cervical third of the upper incisor, the patient has a mild Class II skeletal pattern. If the incisal edge of the lower incisor is anywhere behind this part of the upper there is a gross Class II skeletal pattern.

Similarly, if the adjusted lower incisor impinges on the upper in the incisal third, there is a mild Class III skeletal pattern, if anterior to this a gross Class III skeletal pattern.

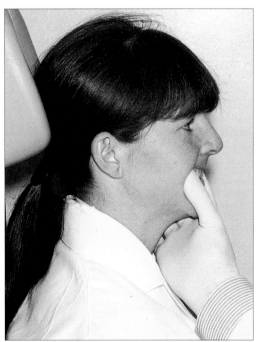

Fig. 4.7 Clinical assessment of upper incisor inclination.

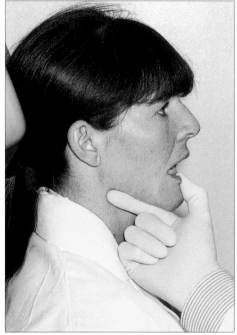

Fig. 4.8 Clinical assessment of lower incisor inclination.

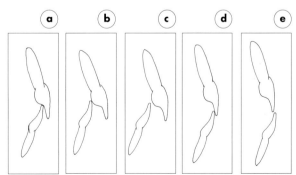

Fig. 4.9 Relationships of mentally adjusted incisors in skeletal I and mild and gross skeletal II and III.
(a) skeletal I (b) mild skeletal II (c) gross skeletal II (d) mild skeletal III (e) gross skeletal III.

There are a few important points about this method:

- It forces the clinician to examine the FM angle and the inclinations of the incisor teeth.
- It is not as complicated, difficult or as inaccurate as it sounds. Frequently, the inclinations of the incisor teeth are found to be normal in which case no mental adjustment is required and the existing overjet can be used to assess the skeletal pattern. In many cases increases or decreases in the FM angle are naturally compensated by proclination or retroclination of lower incisors, so that no mental adjustment is needed.
- Variations in the angle between the crowns and roots of incisor teeth are difficult to assess clinically. Effectively, the method uses the inclination of the crowns of the teeth which can be seen. In some ways, this may be advantageous. This is the aspect of the tooth which is cosmetically important and it is the inclination of the labial surface of the crown which is treated with fixed appliances. It is one of the contradictions of present-day orthodontics that the inclinations of incisor teeth are measured cephalometrically by the long axis and treated to a standard inclination of the labial surface with preadjusted fixed appliances.
- In an individual patient, the occlusion of the teeth as expressed by Angle's classification, is not invariably the same as the skeletal classification due to variations in the position and inclination of the teeth on the jaw bases. Of course, should the skeletal discrepancy be gross, the likelihood is that the occlusal classification will follow the skeletal pattern, but for more minor skeletal discrepancies the two need not necessarily correspond. For example, a mild skeletal III pattern is compatible with a Class II malocclusion (Fig. 4.10).
- The adjustment of incisors to normal inclinations is not necessarily an appropriate treatment. It is well recognised for example that lower incisors will not remain stable if proclined during treatment except in special circumstances.

This instability of lower incisors if proclined or retroclined during treatment leads to a treatment philosophy in which the existing labio-lingual inclinations of lower incisors is accepted and the dentition is rebuilt round this foundation. It also leads to a simplified clinical assessment of the effective skeletal pattern.

The patient is made to sit upright with the Frankfort plane horizontal. The inclination of the upper incisors is assessed and mentally adjusted to normal. If the overjet of these adjusted incisors in relation to the existing positions of the lower incisors is normal, the patient effectively has a normal skeletal pattern and is suitable (in this respect) for simple lingual tipping of upper incisors as might be produced with a removable appliance. If the overjet of the mentally adjusted incisors is greater than normal, other methods will be required.

In a class III malocclusion, the patient is encouraged to bite the incisors edge-to-edge. If this can be achieved without producing a large vertical space between the posterior teeth, the likelihood is that any skeletal discrepancy will not prevent successful treatment by proclining upper incisors, retroclining lower incisors, or both. A large posterior open bite in the edge-to-edge position implies that much proclination of upper and retroclination of lower incisors will be needed to allow the mandible to rotate upwards and the posterior teeth to come into occlusion.

The effect of orthodontic treatment on the profile can not be ignored. The relationship of the lower incisal edge to the A-Po line is easy to measure on cephalometric radiographs but difficult to reproduce clinically. However, a good estimate of the profile can be obtained by placing a straight-edge (conveniently, the edge of a radiograph) against the tip of the nose and soft tissue chin and assessing the position of the lips to this E line (Fig. 4.11). In a young child, the upper lip is ideally on this line and the lower lip just ahead of it. In an adult, where the profile is less convex, the lower lip is ideally on the line with the upper lip just behind it.

Facial growth

The constantly growing face of the child and the long-term nature of orthodontic treatment make prediction of facial growth a desirable goal in orthodontics. Precise prediction is easier said than done. Following development of the cephalostat,[2] early growth studies[3–6] led to the concept that the face grows steadily downwards and forwards in a regular incremental manner along a line, known as the Y or growth axis, joining sella to the chin. If this were so, and if every child grew in an average way, prediction would be easy. Unfortunately, few children who attend for orthodontic treatment have ideal faces and their growth will rarely correspond exactly with average figures. Subsequent studies[7] have shown that during the later stages of growth the profile tends to straighten with the mandible coming further forward than the maxilla.

A later attempt at growth prediction[8] provided simplified forecast grids for five cephalometric points on the assumption that mean annual population growth changes could be applied to individual patients.

Of course, the face presented by the patient at the time of examination represents past growth which may give a useful clue to future growth. Ricketts et al[9] predicted growth by adding to the existing face, growth increments which were appropriate to the age, sex and racial group of the patient in question. This proved

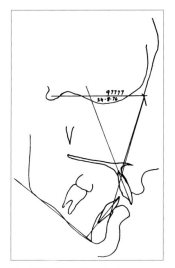

Fig. 4.10 Class II occlusion on mild skeletal III.

quite accurate in patients whose growth was close to the average but was found wanting in those whose growth was more unusual.[10]

Björk[11] proposed a method which predicted the direction of growth rotation of the mandible rather than attempting to predict the future location of cephalometric points quantitatively. Predictive structural features of the mandible were the inclination of the condylar process, curvature of the inferior dental canal, shape of the gonial angle, inclination of the symphysis, the interincisal, interpremolar and intermolar angles and the anterior lower face height. Mandibles with posteriorly inclined condylar processes, inferior dental canals which were nearly a straight line, obtuse gonial angles, anteriorly inclined symphyses and low angles between the upper and lower teeth rotated clockwise during growth (with the patient viewed from the right side) so that the chin moved downward and backward (Fig. 4.12).

Mandibles which had vertical condylar processes, inferior dental canals with a bend in the region of the third molar, low gonial angles, upright symphyseal outlines and high angles between the upper and lower teeth grew more horizontally than vertically with counterclockwise rotation (Fig. 4.13). Maxillae also tended to rotate but to a lesser extent than mandibles.

Some recent work[12,13] has been directed towards distinguishing patients who will fall into certain categories (improve/deteriorate or be stable/unstable) on the basis of discriminant function equations involving large numbers of cephalometric measurements of patients.

Accuracy of prediction ranging from 79% to 100% emerged.

Growth changes in the soft tissue profile, to a limited extent, follow changes in the underlying skeleton. Noses get bigger, profiles become straighter.

Not only the direction and amount but the timing of growth is significant. This has particular importance in the use of functional appliances. Björk[14] has shown that facial growth velocity slows to a prepuberal minimum at about 10 or 11 years and rises to a puberal maximum at about 12 years in girls and 14 years in boys.

Functional appliances seem to have their greatest effect while the face is growing quickly and many clinicians will make serial height measurements of the patient in an attempt to identify the onset of the puberal growth spurt before fitting the appliance. This is not to say that functional appliances are ineffective at other times, but that changes will occur more quickly during a period of active growth. Timing of treatment may be important where there is a risk of expending the compliance of the patient.

Summary

Horizontal and vertical skeletal relationships and the shape of the profile are important in interceptive orthodontics. Most of the significant information can be detected clinically by the practised eye. Prediction of the nature and timing of future facial growth is also useful, particularly if functional appliances are to be used.

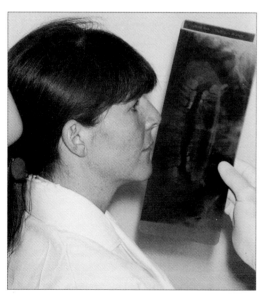

Fig. 4.11 Clinical assessment of the soft tissue profile.

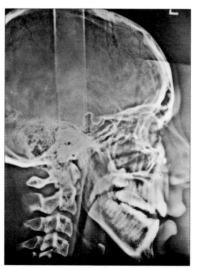

Fig. 4.12 A clockwise rotating mandible.

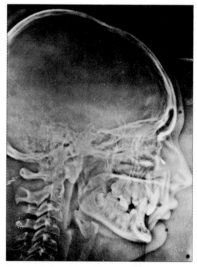

Fig. 4.13 A counterclockwise rotating mandible.

The three key questions in facial growth are:
- In which direction?
- How much?
- When?

This is a rather imprecise science with cephalometric facilities and even less precise without. On the other hand, important information can be gleaned from general trends modified by the existing facial pattern and family likenesses. The average growth of the chin is downwards and forwards. Most mandibles rotate counterclockwise during growth. So do most maxillae but less so. Patients with long faces, oblique jaw angles, poorly developed muscles of mastication and thin mandibular symphyses have mandibles which will rotate clockwise. They are usually tall and slim in body build. Those with short faces, low jaw angles, powerful masseter muscles, broad symphyses and good chin buttons have mandibles which will rotate counterclockwise. They tend to be short and stocky.

Skeletal Class II tends to improve, skeletal Class III tends to deteriorate. There is an average trend for the overbite to diminish during the teenage period. Open bites may improve or deteriorate depending on the aetiology.[15] Open bites with a skeletal element may improve or deteriorate.[16] The computer programme available from the author* will help in prediction of whether an open bite will close spontaneously but a cephalometric radiograph is necessary.

In skeletal Class I cases the orthodontic problem is usually a local factor or space deficiency which is likely to respond to interception. Where there is a Class II or Class III occlusal discrepancy on a skeletal Class I, simple treatment with removable appliances may be sufficient.

The same principle would hold good for minor skeletal Class II and Class III cases where adjustment of the incisor angulation is sufficient to camouflage the skeletal discrepancy. In more substantial Class II skeletal relationships a functional appliance may be indicated at the appropriate age and it may have a favourable effect on the skeletal relationship. In the corresponding Class III skeletal relationship the chincap may be useful.

In general, gross horizontal or vertical skeletal discrepancy cases should be referred to an orthodontist and will probably require surgical correction if the patient is past the age for functional appliances or the chincap.

---

* Outcome prognosis in open bite computed by Andrew Richardson and Terry Gregg.

References

1 Ballard CF. Some bases for aetiology and diagnosis in orthodontics. *Dent Record* 1948; **68**: 133-145.

2 Broadbent BH. A new x-ray technique and its application to orthodontia. *Angle Orthod* 1931; **1**: 45–66 Reprinted *Angle Orthod* 1981; **51**: 93–114.

3 Broadbent BH. The face of the normal child. *Angle Orthod* 1937; **7**: 183–208.

4 Broadbent BH. Bolton standards and technique in orthodontic practice. *Angle Orthod* 1937; **7**: 209–233.

5 Broadbent BH Snr., Broadbent BH Jnr., Golden WH. *Bolton standards of dentofacial developmental growth.* CV Mosby Co. St. Louis 1975.

6 Brodie AG. Some recent observations on the growth of the face and the implications to the orthodontist. *Am J Orthod* 1940; **26**: 741–757.

7 Lande M. Growth behaviour of the human bony profile as revealed by serial cephalometric roentgenology. *Angle Orthod* 1952; **22**: 78–90.

8 Johnston LE. A simplified approach to prediction. *Am J Orthod* 1975; **67**: 253–257.

9 Ricketts RM, Bench RW, Hilgers JJ, Schulhof R. An overview of computerized cephalometrics. *Am J Orthod* 1972; **61**: 1–28.

10 Greenberg LZ, Johnston LE. Computerized prediction: the accuracy of a contemporary long-range forecast. *Am J Orthod* 1975; **67**: 243–252.

11 Björk A. Prediction of mandibular growth rotation. *Am J Orthod* 1969; **55**: 585–599.

12 Finlay J, Richardson A. Outcome prognosis in open bite. *Eur J Orthod* 1995; **17**: 519–523.

13 Battagel JM. The identification of Class III malocclusions by discriminant analysis. *Eur J Orthod* 1994; **16**: 71–80.

14 Björk A. Variations in the growth pattern of the human mandible: longitudinal radiographic study by the implant method. *J Dent Res* 1963; **42**: 400–411.

15 Richardson A. A classification of open bites. *Eur J Orthod* 1981; **3**: 289–296.

16 Richardson A. Facial growth and the prognosis for open bite – a longitudinal study. *Eur Orthod Soc Trans* 1971: 149–157.

17 Brodie AG. Late growth changes in the human face. *Angle Orthod* 1953; **23**:146–157.

18 Björk A. The face in profile. *Svensk Tandl Tidscr* 1947; **40** supp.5B Berlingska Boktryckeriet, Lund.

19 Björk A. The significance of growth changes in the facial pattern and their relationship to changes in occlusion. *Dent Record* 1951; **71**: 197–208.

20 Schulhof RJ, Bagha L. A statistical evaluation of the Ricketts and Johnston growth-forecasting methods. *Am J Orthod* 1975; **67**: 258–276.

21 Björk A, Skieller V. Growth of the maxilla in three dimensions as revealed radiographically by the implant method. *Br J Orthod* 1977; **4**: 53–64.

22 Bhatia SN, Leighton BC. *A manual of facial growth.* Oxford: Oxford University Press 1993.

23 Linder-Aronson S, Woodside DG, Daigle DJ. A longitudinal study of the growth in length of the maxilla in boys between ages 6–20 years. *Eur Orthod Soc Trans* 1975: 169–179.

24 Lundström A, Woodside DG. Individual variation in growth directions expressed at the chin and the midface. *Eur J Orthod* 1980; **2**: 65–79.

25 Lundström A, Woodside DG. A comparison of various facial and occlusal characteristics in mature individuals, with vertical and horizontal growth direction expressed at the chin. *Eur J Orthod* 1981; **3**: 227–235.

26 Lundström A, Woodside DG. Longitudinal changes in facial type in cases with vertical and horizontal growth directions. *Eur J Orthod* 1983; **5**: 259–268.

Summary of evidence for Chapter 4

Topic	Findings	Author/s
X-ray craniometry	Devised cephalostat by modifying craniostat. Almost simultaneous lateral and PA views. Provision for orientating impressions. Stability of cranial base makes it suitable for superimposing films or tracings	Broadbent 1931 (1981).[2] 1700 children between 9 months and 20yrs 'many' x-rayed at six month intervals.
Dento-facial growth	Orderly downward and forward growth of the face except in ill-health. Dental development studied. Described an ugly duckling stage affecting upper incisors, now known as the ugly duckling stage	Broadbent 1937.[3] Longitudinal cephalometric study of more than 1,000 subjects between 9 and 20yrs.
Effect of ill-health on dento-facial growth	Device for orientating impressions abandoned. Tracings of normal and abnormal growth supplied. Growth in pair of twins described. Ill-health affects growth	Broadbent 1937.[4] Individual growth patterns.
Facial growth	Facial shape determined at an early age and thereafter does not change. The nasal area always constitutes 43% of the total face height.	Brodie 1940.[6] Longitudinal cephalometric study of 21 males from 3 months to 8 yrs of age.
Facial growth	Mandible became more prognathic after 7 years. Lower border became more horizontal, horizontal alveolar growth less than basal so facial convexity decreased. No correlation between facial shape at 7 years and subsequent growth.	Lande 1952.[7] Longitudinal cephalometric study of 34 males between 4.4 and 17.1yrs.
Growth prediction	Grids showing annual increments at posterior nasal spine, nose tip, A point, B point and upper molar. Errors similar to errors in identifying cephalometric points on two occasions.	Johnston 1975.[8] Inferred from literature and tested on 19 males and 13 females over 5yrs.
Growth prediction	Computerized laboratory service. Short and long term forecasts of growth with and without treatment.	Ricketts et al 1972.[9] Reports in literature and 2,000 treated cases.
Mandibular growth	Mandibular growth rotation is related to the inclination of condylar and symphyseal processes, shape of the inferior dental canal and gonial angle, face height and angles between upper and lower teeth	Björk 1969.[11] Longitudinal Cephalometric study of 243 Swedish males at 12 and 20yrs and 100 males and females with metallic implants.
Facial growth	Marked consistency and stability of the facial pattern but individual variations existed. Occlusal plane and mandible tend to rotate counter-clockwise. Teeth and alveolar processes become less prominent.	Brodie 1953.[17] Longitudinal cephalometric study of 19 subjects from 8 to 17yrs of age.
Facial growth	On average, prognathism of both jaws increases, mandibular more than maxillary. Overjets and overbites decrease. Incisors become more upright.	Björk 1947.[18] Cephalometric study of 322 Swedish males at 12 and 281 at 20yrs.

Topic (continued)	Findings	Authors
Facial growth	Important individual variations round mean growth pattern. Significance of following individuals longitudinally.	Björk 1951.[19] Longitudinal Cephalometric study of 150 Swedish males at 12 and 20yrs
Forecasting methods compared	Order from least to most accurate: Johnston- averages- Ricketts short-range- Rocky Mountain computer system (devised by Ricketts)	Schulhof & Bagha 1975.[20] Ricketts and Johnston methods tested against averages in 50 cases over 10yrs.
Maxillary growth	Most maxillae rotated counterclockwise but to a lesser extent than mandibles. Nasal floor descended in a parallel manner in relation to cranial base. Zygomatic process stable in relation to implants.	Björk & Skieller 1977.[21] Longitudinal cephalometric study of 9 males with implants from 4 to 21yrs of age.
Facial growth	Distance and velocity growth curves of age changes in over 300 linear and angular dental, skeletal, and soft tissue parameters. Annual growth profiles give quantitative description of facial growth used as baseline research data and in clinical orthodontics	Bhatia & Leighton 1993.[22]
Maxillary growth	Large individual variations in growth velocity. No appreciable prepuberal acceleration. No relation with growth in stature	Linder-Aronson et al 1975.[23] Longitudinal cephalometric study of 62M in Burlington from 6-20yrs. (38 treated before age 10yrs)
Growth at chin and midface	More horizontal growth at chin and midface in males. Very few backward growing mandibles in Burlington which may be related to airway or recovery from treatment which extruded molars	Lundström & Woodside 1980.[24] Longitudinal cephalometric study of 109F,117M in Burlington from 3–20yrs (48% treated) and 40F,60M in Ann Arbor
Mature face	Vertical growers showed greater facial height, more retrognathic chin, steeper mandibular plane, larger gonial angle, less cranial base flexure	Lundström & Woodside 1981.[25] Same material as above
Prediction of growth direction	Mandibular retrognathism measurable at 9yrs and wide cranial base angle increased in vertical growers. Counter-clockwise rotation of mandibular plane in horizontal growers	Lundström & Woodside 1983.[26] Same material as above

Soft tissue morphology, behaviour and maturation

The evidence-based findings are summarised on pages 38 and 39.

In orthodontic terminology, the 'soft tissues' may be taken to mean all non-calcified structures which are relevant to tooth positions and orthodontic treatment. These include the lips, tongue and cheeks, the floor of the mouth, the palate and throat and associated musculature. The principal muscle groups involved are muscles of mastication and facial expression and the intrinsic and extrinsic muscles of the tongue. The term may also embrace the gums and periodontal ligaments although they are not intrinsically mobile.

An exception is made of the labial fraenum which may be associated with a diastema and is considered under the heading of local irregularities in Chapter 8.

Lips

At birth, the shape of the vermilion borders of the lips is almost round. During the first two years of life the width of the mouth doubles while the height diminishes, thus converting a sphincter suitable for suckling into a slit. During adolescence, annual changes amounting to less than 0.5mm are much less dramatic. The lower lip becomes more protrusive and more convex, whereas the changes in the upper lip are more variable, some becoming more convex and others flattening.[1]

During growth and development, lip growth exceeds vertical growth of the lower face.[2] In consequence, lips tend to become more competent with the lower lip covering more of the upper incisors.[3] However, there is a transient stage during the eruption of the incisors and first molars when the lips are particularly incompetent.[4] Lip growth usually diminishes to an imperceptible level at 13 years in females but continues to about 18 years in males.[5]

In males, the upper lip descends in relation to the upper incisors. Attempts to correlate lip changes with late crowding of lower incisors have produced inconclusive results.[6]

The classification of lip morphology is borrowed from sphincters elsewhere in the body. They may be competent (able to close), incompetent or potentially competent.

Competent lips (Fig. 5.1) are defined as that condition in which the lips at rest meet to form an anterior oral seal with the mandible in the rest position. Incompetent lips (Fig. 5.2) are those which do not meet under the same conditions.

In theory, the cause of lip incompetence may be anything producing a disproportion between the length of the lips and the distance to be spanned, e.g. short lips, a long face or a gross horizontal skeletal discrepancy. This theory presupposes that the length of the lips and the skeletal framework are inherited as independent variables. Research has failed to demonstrate a relationship between the muscular contraction in producing a lip seal and face height. Incompetence is, however, correlated with the horizontal skeletal pattern and overjet.[7]

Potentially competent lips (Fig. 5.3) are those

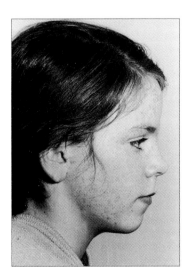
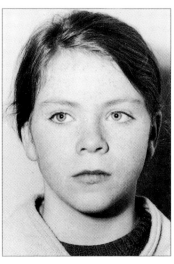

Fig. 5.1 Competent lips.

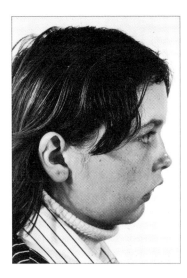
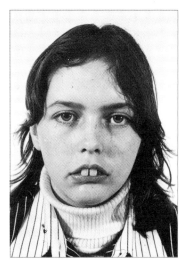

Fig. 5.2 Incompetent lips.

which are long enough to span the space between the jaws but are prevented from doing so by the interposition of the upper incisor teeth. Following treatment of the increased overjet, potentially competent lips become competent.

Electromyographic and pressure transducer studies have both demonstrated that intermittent lip pressures during chewing, swallowing and speech are poorly correlated with tooth positions. On the other hand, there is evidence that the almost constant pressures exerted by the lips and cheeks in the habitual posture have an influence on tooth positions.[8,9] In terms of the effect on the dentition the distinction between competent lips and incompetent lips is important but the degree of incompetence, judged electromyographically, is not. When the lips are competent, there is a relationship between 'resting' perioral activity and tooth positions.[9]

There can be no question that holding the lips and cheeks away from the teeth with an appliance results in wider and less crowded arches. In clinical orthodontics, the real question is what happens when the appliance is removed. Followers of the equilibration theory say that relapse is inevitable, but Fränkel and Fränkel demonstrate cases treated with the Function Regulator appliance which show remarkable stability many years out of retention.[10]

The habitual position of the lower lip in relation to the upper incisors is very important. Normally, the lower lip covers the incisal one third of the labial surface of the upper incisors.

In patients whose lower lip lies below or behind the incisal edges of the upper incisors, the overjet is usually increased. When the lower lip lies in front of the upper incisors, the overjet may be normal or reduced depending on the skeletal pattern and the position of the incisal edges of the lower incisors.

Sealing of the lips anterior to the labial surfaces of retracted upper incisors contributes to stability.[11]

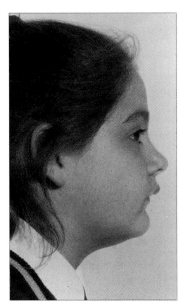
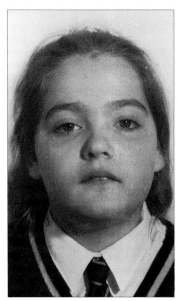

Fig. 5.3 Potentially competent lips.

Especially where the lower lip is tight and 'strap-like', proclination of lower incisors with an appliance will not be stable. Interceptive treatment of lower arch crowding by premolar or first molar extractions without appliance therapy should be avoided in these cases for fear that the lower incisors will tilt lingually.

Tongue

The interesting features of the tongue are the size, resting position and function in swallowing and speech. Reproducible measurement of tongue size in two dimensions is possible on cephalometric radiographs providing the position of the mandible is limited to a small range. Large tongue areas measured on cephalometric films are associated with proclination of the incisor teeth and small tongue areas with retroclination. After the age of 13 years, the area of the tongue increases more than the area of the intermaxillary space.[12]

Low tongue resting postures are found in subjects with Class III malocclusions and crossbites, high tongue resting postures in Class II division 2 malocclusion and scissors bites.

Where there is nasal obstruction and mouth-breathing, the lower face is long, the tongue has a low resting position, the upper arch is narrow and the incisors are retroclined.[13] The lower incisors procline spontaneously following adenoidectomy and the consequent altered mode of breathing and head posture.[14]

Some patients with Class II division 1 malocclusions on Class II skeletal patterns will produce an anterior oral seal between the tongue and lower lip which is often associated with an incomplete overbite.

The swallowing behaviour in an infant is with the jaws separated and the tongue protruded. The normal swallowing behaviour in an adult is with the teeth together, the tongue contained within the dental arches and little or no contraction of the circumoral musculature.[15] Children usually change from the infantile to the adult behaviour sometime between 2 and 5 years but some individuals never change and maintain a tooth-apart swallow with a tongue thrust throughout life.

Tongue thrusting behaviour is associated with an anterior open bite and is quite common in young children (Fig. 5.4). Providing the abnormality of tongue behaviour is not very vigorous, the open bite is likely to close of its own accord. Much more sinister is the so-called endogenous tongue thrust which is part of the neuromuscular make-up of the child and will remain with the patient throughout life.

The behaviour of the soft tissues is partly hereditary and partly acquired. Most of the skills of speech are acquired. The infant cry at birth is followed by the articulation of simple words at about 6 months and by an extended vocabulary of disconnected words before 12 months. Between 18 months and 2 years a series of words is joined together.

Most children seem to cope with the changing environment of the mouth cavity as teeth erupt and are shed without undue difficulty but an interdental sigmatism or lisp is quite a common developmental feature. In the vast majority of children the pattern of soft tissue behaviour matures but the combination of a vigorous tongue thrust on swallowing and a lisp is a traditional warning sign to the orthodontist that tooth positions will not improve spontaneously and that treatment results are likely to relapse. Cases where the soft tissue function is a serious impediment to orthodontic treatment are rare, amounting to 1.35% in one sample.[16]

Muscles of mastication

The size and activity of the muscles of mastication have a direct effect on the development of bony muscular processes to which they are attached and an indirect effect on the positions of the teeth through the inclined planes of intercuspation. In relation to forces generated by muscles of the lips and cheeks, the forces of mastication are very high, but they are applied much less frequently.

Where the cusps are high and the interdigitation is deep, the forces of occlusion tend to maintain the relationship of the teeth but, since the teeth are somewhat mesially inclined, there is a mesially directed resolved part of the force

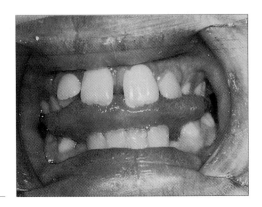

Fig. 5.4 Tongue thrusting.

of mastication which is often called the anterior component of force. This mesially directed force may contribute to the forward movement of the dentition and associated crowding of anterior teeth. In general, the stabilising forces of interdigitation can be easily overcome in moving teeth with orthodontic appliances but movement of teeth in one arch may induce corresponding movement of the opposing teeth.[17] Occasionally, upper arch expansion in cases of crossbite does not move the upper teeth which are in lingual occlusion but produces a scissors bite of the teeth on the other side. Such problems may be overcome by adding anterior or posterior bite planes to the appliance.

During growth and development, the muscles of mastication become more bulky and their areas of bony attachment more extensive. The Temporalis spreads vertically and antero-posteriorly along the side of the skull and the Masseter and Medial pterygoid achieve broad attachments to the angle of the mandible. These areas of attachment may show prominent ridging and lipping of the bone in races indulging in masticatory athleticism such as gnawing bones, which is common in Africa, or chewing leather boots to soften them, as prac-tised by Esquimaux women.

Associated with the change in size of muscles as the child develops, there is a change in function with the Temporalis predominating in the child and the Masseter in the adult.[18]

In a patient with normal occlusion, there is balanced activity of the muscles of mastication with synchronous onset of muscle activity in mandibular movements. When the jaw relationship is abnormal in the lateral or antero-posterior direction the muscles seem to be actively engaged in attempts to normalise the jaw relationship. When there is a displacement due to cuspal interference, the muscular activity is similar to a patient with normal occlusion deliberately biting in a displaced position.

Patients with anterior open bite and a steeply angled occlusal plane have poorly developed muscles of mastication and low muscular activity. Patients with a more horizontal occlusal plane as in Class II division 2 mal-occlusion have high muscular activity and a broad mandibular ramus.[19,20]

Periodontium

Connective tissue fibres of the periodontal liga-ment and gum surrounding the roots of teeth are an important factor in maintaining tooth positions. If a tooth is moved orthodontically, there is a tendency for the adjacent tooth to move with it due to the connection of transseptal fibres. If these fibres are cut repeatedly to prevent healing, the connection between the teeth is lost and they drift apart.[21] When a tooth is extracted, the contraction of scar tissue across the socket tends to close the space. Similarly, a fraenectomy alone will often be followed by spontaneous closure of an upper midline diastema.

Resistance of the gingival crest fibres to stretching may impede orthodontic tooth movement. This may be a particular problem when teeth are being rotated because all fibrous attachments are stretched as distinct from simple mesial or distal movement when only half of the fibres are in tension.[22] The general statement is that rotations of teeth are difficult to maintain but this is not universally true. Rotations associated with crowding do not present problems if the crowding is adequately treated. It is rotations where the teeth are spaced (so-called idiopathic rotations) which can be troublesome. These may be treated by over-derotating the tooth supplemented by pericision, a technique in which the supra-alveolar fibres are cut with a fine blade.[23, 24] Alternatively or additionally, a permanent retainer can be used.

During the 1960s there was a preoccupation with the soft tissues of the lips, cheeks and tongue in British orthodontics. The thesis was that the teeth were in a position of balance between forces exerted by the lips and cheeks on the outside of the arch and those exerted by the tongue on the inside. The term 'soft tissue balance' always seemed a misnomer because the other forces acting on the teeth were ignored, and subsequent work showed that tongue pressure usually exceeds lip pressure.[25, 26]

Nonetheless, it is reasonable to conclude that the presence of the lower lip between upper and lower incisors contributes to maintenance of an increased overjet, and that excessive contrac-tion of the mentalis and suprahyoid groups of muscles in producing an anterior oral seal between incompetent lips produces an impedi-ment to tooth movement. Muscle training exer-cises were popular in the 1930s [27] and were fashionable in the 1950s. General present-day opinion in this country is that there is little scope for intercepting abnormalities of the soft tissue morphology and function by muscle training, but it must be said that a number of orthodontists believe that exercises and appli-ances which stimulate or educate muscles can change unfavourable influences into favourable ones.[10]

The study of soft tissue morphology and function is a somewhat imprecise science and clinical application of the findings even more so. The following guidelines are offered as clinical working hypotheses:

- Proclination of lower incisors in class I or class II cases is usually unstable except when the incisors are deeply trapped behind the palate or upper incisors and the overbite can be reduced, or where there is a habit which is abandoned.
- A 'strap-like' lower lip which intrudes between the upper and lower incisors will be an impediment to proclination of lower incisors or retroclination of upper incisors. Treatment of lower arch crowding by extraction without appliance therapy should be avoided in these cases. Likewise, extraction of upper teeth without appliance therapy will not result in overjet reduction.

- The stability of upper incisors which have been retracted mechanically depends, to an extent, on having the lower lip resting anterior to their labial surfaces.
- Lateral arch expansion in the fully developed dentition is rarely stable.
- If there is proclination and spacing of the incisors, an anterior open bite with a vigorous tongue thrust on swallowing and a lisp, the prospects for stable correction are not good.
- The occlusion of the teeth is rarely an impediment to tooth movement. If it is troublesome, use a bite plane.
- Stable derotation of spaced teeth is problematic. It may be enhanced by overderotation, pericision and permanent retention.

References

1 Burke PH. Serial growth changes in the lips. *Br J Orthod* 1980; **7**: 17–30.

2 Vig PS, Cohen AM. Vertical growth of the lips: A serial cephalometric study. *Am J Orthod* 1979; **75**: 405–415.

3 Jackson D. Lip positions and incisor relationships. *Br Dent J* 1962; **112**: 147–155.

4 Moss JP, Picton DCA. The problems of dental development among children on a Greek island. *Dent Practit* 1968; **18**: 442–448.

5 Nanda RS, Meng H, Kapila S, Goorhuis J. Growth changes in the soft tissue facial profile. *Angle Orthod* 1990; **60**: 177–190.

6 Richardson ME. Late lower arch crowding in relation to soft tissue maturation. *Am J Orthod Dentofac Orthop* 1997; **112**: 159–164.

7 Simpson M McF. Lip competence and its relationship to skeletal and dental morphology – an electromyographic investigation. *Br J Orthod* 1976; **3**: 177–179.

8 Profitt WR, Fields HW. *Contemporary Orthodontics*. 2nd Ed. St Louis: Mosby Year Book 1993.

9 Harradine NWT, Kirchen RHES. Lip and mentalis activity and its influence on incisor position – a quantitative electromyographic study. *Br J Orthod* 1983; **10**: 114–127.

10 Fränkel R, Fränkel C. *Orofacial orthopedics with the function regulator*. Basel: Karger 1993.

11 Orton HS. Some cases showing deliberate labial movement of the upper incisor apices during the reduction of the overjet with special reference to lip behaviour. *Dent Practit* 1966; **17**: 97–105.

12 Cohen AM, Vig PS. A serial growth study of the tongue and intermaxillary space. *Angle Orthod* 1976; **46**: 332–337.

13 Linder-Aronson S. Adenoids, their effect on the mode of breathing and nasal air flow and their relationship to characteristics of the facial skeleton and the dentition. *Acta Oto-laryng* 1970; Supplementum: 265.

14 Linder-Aronson S, Woodside DG, Hellsing E, Emerson W. Normalisation of incisor position after adenoidectomy. *Am J Orthod Dentofac Orthoped* 1993; **103**: 412–427.

15 Ardran GM, Kemp FH. A radiographic study of movements of the tongue in swallowing. *Dent Practit* 1955; **5**: 252–261.

16 Tulley WJ. The tongue: that unruly member. *Dent Practit* 1964; **15**: 27–38.

17 Elder JR, Tuenge RH. Cephalometric and histological changes produced by extra-oral high pull traction to the maxilla in macaca mulatta. *Am J Orthod* 1974; **66**: 559–644.

18 Moss JP, Chalmers CP. An electromyographic investigation of patients with a normal jaw relationship and a Class III jaw relationship. *Am J Orthod* 1974; **66**: 538–556.

19 Moss, JP. The soft tissue environment of the teeth and jaws Experimental malocclusion: parts 2 and 3. *Br J Orthod* 1980; **7**: 205–216.

20 Raadsheer MC, van Eijden TMJG, van Ginkel FC, Prahl-Andersen B. Contribution of jaw muscle size and craniofacial morphology to human bite force magnitude. *J Dent Res* 1999; **78**: 31–42.

21 Moss JP, Picton DCA. The effect on approximal drift of cheek teeth of dividing mandibular molars of adult monkeys (Macaca Irus) *Arch Oral Biol* 1974; **19**: 1211–1214.

22 Edwards JG. A study of the periodontium during orthodontic rotation of teeth. *Am J Orthod* 1968; **54**: 441–461.

23 Edwards JG. A surgical procedure to eliminate rotational relapse. *Am J Orthod* 1970; **57**: 35–46.

24 Pinson PR, Strahan JD. The effect on the relapse of orthodontically rotated teeth of surgical division of the gingival fibres pericision. *Br J Orthod* 1974; **1**: 87–91.

25 Gould MSE, Picton DCA. A method of measuring forces acting on the teeth from the lips, cheeks and tongue. *Br Dent J* 1962; **112**: 235–242.

26 Luffingham JK. Soft tissue pressure and dental arch form. *Eur Orthod Soc Trans* 1969: 313–328.

27 Chapman H. Exercises. Abnormalities of position: treatment. In Bennett Sir N (ed.). *The science and practice of dental surgery*. pp 589–596. London: Waverley, 1931.

28 Farkas LG, Katic BA, Hreczko TA, Deutch C, Munro IR. Anthropometric proportions in the upper lip-lower lip-chin area of the lower face in young white adults. *Am J Orthod* 1984; **86**: 52–60.

Summary of evidence for Chapter 5

Topic	Findings	Author/s
Soft tissue morphology	Birth to 1yr: large lateral increase in lips, diminution in vertical size. At adolescence: lower lip becomes more convex and protrusive, upper lip flattens.	Burke 1980[1]. Stereophotogrammetry of a baby from 3weeks to 2yrs and 6 pairs of like-sexed twins over adolescence.
Lip growth	Lips grow up to 19yrs. Lip growth exceeds growth in anterior facial height.	Vig & Cohen 1979[2]. Longitudinal cephalometric study of 50 subjects between 4 and 20yrs.
Soft tissue growth	Largest increase in nose. Nose still growing at 18yrs in males. Length of upper lip complete by 15yrs both sexes. Lips get longer and thicker in males than females.	Nanda et al. 1990 [5]. Longitudinal cephalometric study of 23F,17M from 7 to 18yrs.
Lip morphology and incisor crowding	Cross-sectional area of lips increased, lip separation reduced especially in males. Upper lip descended in males.	Richardson ME 1997[6]. Longitudinal cephalometric study of 23F, 23M between 12.5 and 15.5yrs.
Lip incompetence	Mentalis and suprahyoid group most active in lip seal. Activity correlates with overjet and ANB angle. Upper lip activity correlates with interincisal angle.	Simpson 1976[7]. Cephalometry and electro myography of 17F,4M with incompetent lips in lip seal.
Muscle activity in relation to incisor position	Perioral activity not influenced by lip competence. Incisor positions determined by resting perioral activity in competent subjects. Intermittent activity has no significance.	Harradine & Kirchen 1983[9]. 41 subjects with Class II malocclusions. EMG of masseter, upper lip, lower lip and mentalis in speech, lip seal, swallow and chewing.
Growth of tongue and intermaxillary space	Tongue becomes relatively larger. Growth continues longer in males. Increase in tongue size perhaps compensated by descent.	Cohen & Vig 1976[12]. Longitudinal cephalometric study of 25F,25M.
Adenoids and facial and dental form	In adenoidectomy group more frequent narrow upper arch, crossbite, retroclination of incisors, large face height.	Linder-Aronson 1970[13]. Cast, cephalometric and airflow study of 81 for adenoidectomy and 81 normals matched for sex, age.
Effect of airway on incisor inclinations	Changed mode of breathing after adenoidectomy associated with labial movement of incisor teeth.	Linder-Aronson et al 1993[14]. Longitudinal cephalometric study of 16F,22M with adenoidectomy compared with 17F,20M untreated.
Swallowing	When swallowing fluid or small lumps of solids, tongue is thrust forward against upper incisor teeth, mandible is elevated.	Ardran & Kemp 1955[15]. Cineradiographic study of 250 adults swallowing.

Topic (continued)	Findings	Author/s
Muscle activity	Intercuspal was the best position for discrimination between groups. There was a more normal pattern of activity after treatment.	Moss & Chalmers 1974[18]. EMG of Masseter and Temporalis in intercuspal, protruded and retruded positions. 40 with normal occlusion, 15 with skeletal III, 15 with postural class III, 30 after treatment.
Muscle activity	Muscular attempts to normalise jaw relationships. Low muscular activity in open bite, high muscular activity in Class II div.2.	Moss 1980[19]. Electromyography of 30 with mandibular prognathism, 38 with unilateral hyperplasia, 20 with deviations, 10 with skeletal open bite and 10 with Class II div.2.
Maximal bite force, muscle size and facial morphology	Bite force varies positively with thickness of masseter, vertical and transverse facial size and inclination of midface, negatively with inclination of occlusal plane and mandible.	Raadsheer et al 1999[20]. Maximal bite forces, cephalometry, anthropometrics and ultrasonography of 63F,58M adults.
Transseptal fibres and approximal drift	Tooth fragments moved together on experimental side, separated on control side due to contraction of intact transseptal fibre system.	Moss & Picton 1974[21]. Spaces created between teeth in 7 monkeys. Some molars divided vertically. Interdental soft tissues removed every 2 weeks on experimental side. Distances between amalgam fillings measured.
Effect of rotation with appliances on the gingivae	Line of marks bent in the direction of rotation. After 5 months retention, marks had not straightened and gingival and transseptal fibres were still taut.	Edwards 1968[22]. In 6 dogs and 4 volunteer patients, a vertical line of marks was tattooed into the gingivae relating to teeth before rotation with appliances.
Effect of pericision	Tattoo line bent in direction of rotation. Relapse occurred in 8 teeth where arches were removed and they were retreated. Following surgery, tattoo line straightened within 40 hours. Negligible relapse up to 3 months following surgery.	Edwards 1970[23]. 12 patients had tattoo marks before rotations of 16 teeth. Arches were removed from 8. Subsequently, all 16 were pericised to 3mm below the alveolar bone crest.
Effect of pericision	Significantly less relapse in pericised teeth (25.5% of original) as against non-pericised teeth (56.5% of original). Between 16 and 28 weeks retention is appropriate.	Pinson & Strahan[24]. Relapse of 21 derotated and pericised teeth compared with 10 derotated teeth without pericision at least 1 year out of retention.
Soft tissue pressures	During swallowing and speech peak pressures much greater on lingual side. Pressures in resting posture quite small.	Luffingham 1969[26]. Buccal and lingual pressures measured with sensors in 9 subjects.
Lip and chin proportions	Upper lip occupies 1/3 of lower face, lower lip more than 1/3. Skin covers 73.5% of the upper lip in males, 68% in females and 63% of the lower lip in males and 61.1% in females	Farkas et al[28]. Anthropometric measurements of 39F,50M Caucasian hospital employees and 50F,50M students.

6 Early interceptive treatment

The evidence-based findings are summarised on page 49.

In the course of growth and development of the child, the rest position (or endogenous postural position) of the mandible precedes the eruption of teeth. It is said to be present by the third month of life and to be still present even if all the teeth are extracted in later life.[1] The inviolable nature of the rest position of the mandible, which is dictated by the resting length of muscles and ligaments, is derived from its importance in essential functions such as respiration and swallowing. It is into the intermaxillary space dictated by the rest position and centric relation of the jaws that the teeth and alveolar processes grow and the occlusion of the teeth is established.

The moment the first pair of upper and lower teeth make occlusal contact there will exist two factors (the muscles and the teeth) influencing the mandible in its functional range of movement. Ideally, the range of mandibular movement dictated by the muscles should be in harmony with that dictated by the teeth. Unfortunately, this does not always occur. Where there is a discrepancy between muscular positioning and the jaw relationship determined by the teeth, the jaws are not in centric relation when the teeth are in occlusion and the patient will show a displacement or deflection of the mandible in closing from the rest position. These displacements may be anterior, lateral or posterior.

Anterior displacements

Anterior displacements (Fig. 6.1) may be present where the upper incisors bite on the lingual side of their lower counterparts. These anomalies are best treated at an early stage because the labial surfaces of the upper incisors may be abraded by the lowers, the periodontal support of the incisors may suffer as a result of occlusal trauma and elimination of the displacement will promote establishment of centric relationship. Left untreated, the Class III incisor relationship will tend to produce further retroclination of upper incisors and proclination of lower incisors, accentuating the discrepancy. Thus, an early postural class III incisor relationship becomes an established malocclusion. In addition, early correction of the displacement will allow the teeth which erupt later to come into occlusion on the foundation of the correct jaw relationship.

The most popular treatment of upper incisors in lingual occlusion is an upper removable appliance, with cantilever springs in 0.5mm wire, incorporating molar capping to separate the upper and lower incisor teeth (Fig. 6.2). A single cantilever spring is adequate for the proclination of 1 tooth. If more than 1 tooth is to be proclined a double cantilever spring is preferable because equal forces can be exerted on both teeth by adjusting both coils (Fig. 6.3). The spring is held in position against the incisor

(a)

(b)

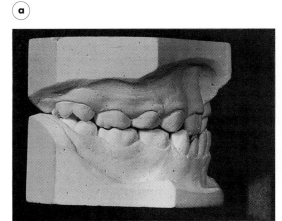
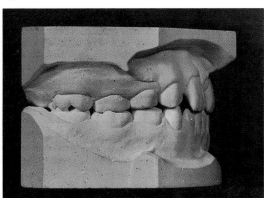

Fig. 6.1 (a) Anterior displacement with upper incisors in lingual occlusion. (b) after proclination of incisors. Note the changed relationship of the deciduous canines and first permanent molars.

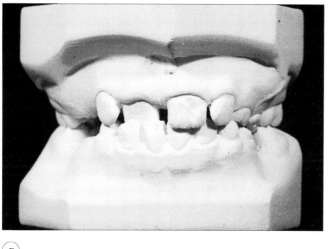

(a)

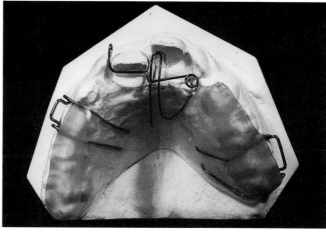

(b)

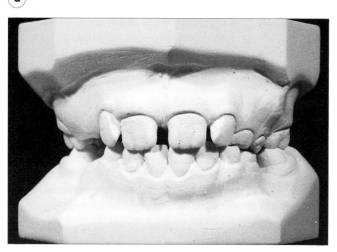

(c)

Fig. 6.2 Lingual occlusion of an upper central incisor. (a) before treatment (b) upper removable appliance with single cantilever spring (c) after treatment.

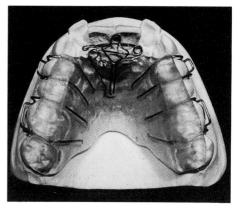

Fig. 6.3 Removable appliance to correct lingual occlusion of more than one upper incisor. Double cantilever spring with arrowhead guard.

teeth with a wire guard. Successive adjustments of the spring soon take it beyond the control of the guard and there is a tendency for the patient to wear the spring on the wrong side of the guard so that the spring is held away from the tooth. The effective length of the guard can be increased by cranking the spring, as in Figure 6.2, or by making the guard in the form of an arrowhead (see Fig. 6.3). The tip of the arrowhead can be moved labially by squeezing the arrowhead with universal pliers.

Since the active part of the appliance bears against the sloping palatal surface of the incisor or incisors at the front of the mouth, there is a tendency for the anterior end of the appliance to be displaced downwards. The customary placement of Adams clasps on partially erupted first permanent molars may be too remote from the area of displacement to be fully effective, and it is important to improve retention by placing additional clasps on the first deciduous molars if they are still firm. It has been pointed out that the molar capping is not strictly necessary and simply increases the bulk of the appliance, leading to problems with

patient compliance. While the appliance will be effective without separating the teeth, the capping is easily incorporated as an extension of the baseplate and it ensures that upper incisors can be aligned without a period of traumatic occlusion as they move from the lingual to the labial side of the lower incisors. In the author's experience, the additional bulk does not seem to trouble patients.

One difficulty with the molar capping is that it reduces the flexibility of the Adams clasps if the approximal part of the clasps are contained in the acrylic resin. The solution is to exclude the acrylic from these areas by plastering them out before heat-curing the baseplate or by waxing them out if a cold-cure resin is used (Fig. 6.4).

In many cases, "popping an incisor over the bite" is not as simple as the term might indicate. The prudent practitioner will run through the following checklist before commencing treatment:

• The Class III skeletal discrepancy should not be so gross that the incisor relationship cannot be corrected without over-proclining upper incisors. In patients who have an anterior displacement, it is sometimes difficult to judge how much of the apparent basal discrepancy is truly skeletal and how much is due to the displacement. A useful test, described in Chapter 4, is to determine whether the incisor teeth can be brought edge-to-edge, as though biting a piece of thread. If an edge-to-edge relationship can be achieved without producing a large vertical space between the posterior teeth, the prognosis for treatment is good. The size of the vertical space between the posterior teeth is rarely mentioned when conducting this test, yet it is important because a great deal of proclination of incisors may be needed to allow the posterior teeth to come into occlusion.

- The overbite at the end of treatment should be sufficient to maintain the corrected incisor relationship.
- There should be sufficient space between the deciduous canines to permit proclination of the incisors. If not, consideration should be given to extracting both deciduous canines to make space, preserving the mid-line at the same time.
- There is frequently an abnormal relationship of the upper and lower deciduous canines which will maintain a forward displacement even after correction of the incisor relationship. It is important to treat this displacement by grinding or extraction of the deciduous canines.
- The position of the unerupted maxillary canine should be confirmed by palpation and radiological investigation if necessary. Particularly in narrow upper arches, the permanent canine often develops in a forward position over the buccal side of the lateral incisor (Fig. 6.5). There is a danger that proclination of the lateral incisor will move it against the follicle of the canine, leading to resorption of the lateral incisor root. In these cases, it is better to await eruption of the canine and move it distally before proclination of the lateral incisor is attempted. This is one of the very few instances when correction of a single incisor in lingual occlusion should be delayed. Care should also be exercised when the canine is in an ectopic palatal position. In this case, the canine will be at a higher level near the apex of the lateral incisor and is notoriously associated with apical resorption of the lateral incisor. Proclination of the lateral incisor with a removable appliance will move the apex in a palatal direction which will accelerate the resorption process. Treatment decisions in these cases depend on what is to be done with the ectopic canine.

- Anterior crossbites are often regarded as antero-posterior malocclusions, but there is frequently a superadded lateral complication leading to an upper arch which is too narrow to match the lower. In these cases, proclining a palatally placed upper lateral incisor and achieving sufficient overbite in relation to a big, bulbous, buccally placed lower canine can be problematical. This difficulty is best met by moving the lower canine distally and lingually before, or at the same time as, the upper lateral is being proclined. This is another exception to the rule of early treatment.

- The final problem is growth. Most orthodontists will have found themselves proclining upper incisors in cases where deterioration in the skeletal relationship is sufficiently rapid that little progress is made. Important clues to this kind of growth pattern may be found in careful examination of the facial and dental relationships described in Chapter 4 and in parents and older siblings. When in doubt, it is wise to monitor growth for some time before commencing treatment.

Some orthodontists treat lingual occlusion of all the upper incisors with a functional appliance.[2,3] In the hands of the author, functional appliances work less well in Class III malocclusions than in Class II because it is more difficult to take an over-retruded bite than one which is protruded.

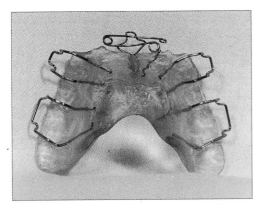

Fig. 6.4 Boxing out the crossovers of Adams clasps. Palatal view of the appliance showing the crossovers of the clasps free of the acrylic over the occlusal surfaces of the teeth.

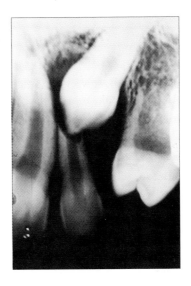

Fig. 6.5 Maxillary canine resorbing the root of a lateral incisor.

A third treatment possibility is the chin cap with extra-oral traction (Fig. 6.6). Some authorities believe that this appliance is capable of restraining mandibular growth, while others maintain that the principal effect lies in retrocli-nation of the lower incisors.[4] It has been shown that the lower permanent incisors are almost invariably more retroclined before eruption than after eruption.[5,6] Wearing a chincap at the crucial time during early eruption may prevent

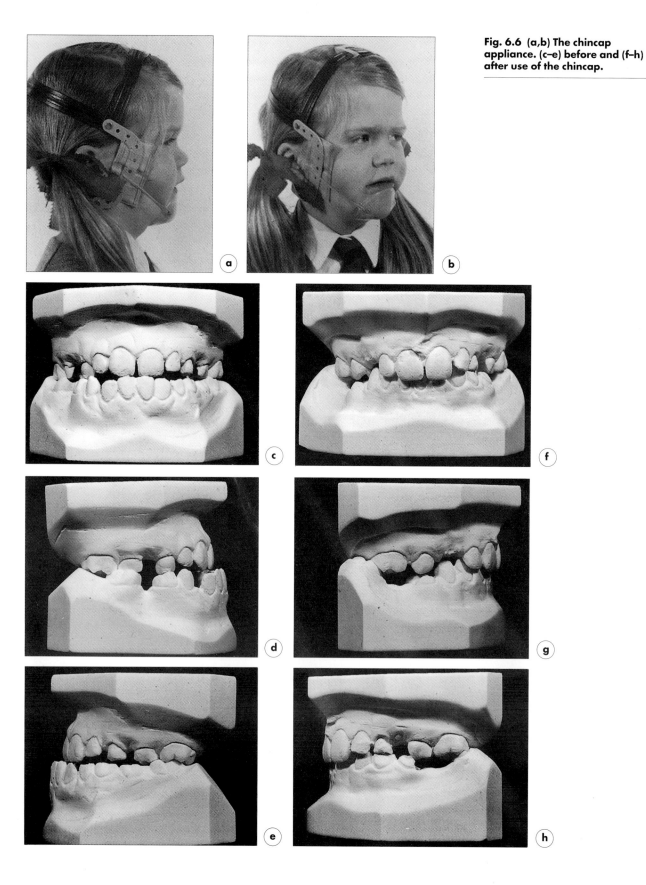

Fig. 6.6 (a,b) The chincap appliance. (c–e) before and (f–h) after use of the chincap.

the usual spontaneous proclination of these teeth. Recent work has confirmed that the chincap retroclines lower incisors and redirects mandibular growth in a vertical rather than a horizontal direction, together with marked improvement in the soft tissue profile.[7] Chincap therapy may be combined with an appliance to procline upper incisors where it is appropriate. The indications for the chincap combined with an upper removable appliance are a child aged 7–9 years with a Class III malocclusion, diminished lower face height, proclined lower incisors and upper incisors which are not already proclined. Recent research has shown that early correction of the incisor relationship may allow later discrepancies in skeletal growth to be compensated for, or camouflaged by, further spontaneous proclination of upper and retroclination of lower incisors if the overbite is substantial.[8] On the other hand, should the skeletal relationship deteriorate with growth and surgery become inevitable, the orthodontic preparation for surgery will involve adjustment of incisor inclinations to normal values thus reversing the initial treatment. This is the clinical enigma in these cases. Patients after chincap treatment are delighted with their facial appearance and diminution in teasing by their peers at a sensitive time in their lives. In addition, it is important for them to feel that something is being done. This constitutes an important psychosocial service to patients as pointed out by Profitt and White.[9]

It is a matter of clinical judgement whether chincap therapy is appropriate for each individual patient.

Lateral displacements

There are some posterior crossbites of the deciduous dentition which are associated with a habit of thumb sucking. These crossbites tend to be corrected spontaneously on eruption of the permanent teeth, providing the habit is abandoned. The problem is that these spontaneous corrections occur in less than half of the number of cases seen and their occurrence is difficult to predict.[10] In deciding which patients to treat and which to leave in the expectation of spontaneous improvement, it is best to be guided by the severity of the crossbite, treating only the more severe. In the same way as anterior displacements, lateral displacements may be accentuated by the crossbite of the rather long and unworn deciduous canines which require treatment by grinding or extraction. If occlusal grinding or extraction of deciduous canines alone will not suffice, such lateral crossbites and displacements may be treated by upper arch expansion by an orthodontist. Gaining retention for a removable appliance on deciduous molars may be difficult, and quite precise activation of the appliance is needed to prevent dislodgement. Figure 6.7 shows a girl whose upper deciduous arch was expanded in association with grinding of the deciduous canines and who subsequently developed a good occlusion.

Posterior displacements

Posterior displacements are the most difficult to detect but may provoke the most severe symptoms. They may arise early in a skeletal II environment where the line of eruption of the teeth and the balance of forces round the incisors is such that the upper (and sometimes the lower) incisors become retroclined. Because of the large angle between the upper and lower incisors there are no incisal occlusal stops, the incisors continue erupting and the overbite

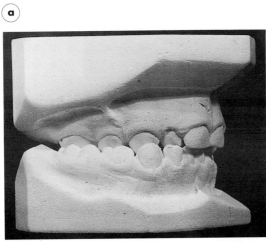
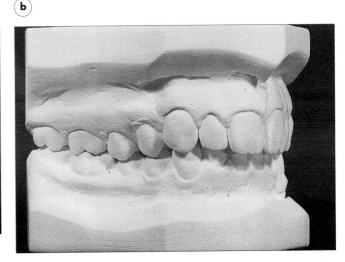

Fig. 6.7 Correction of crossbite by arch expansion and grinding of deciduous canines. (a) aged 4 years, (b) aged 13 years.

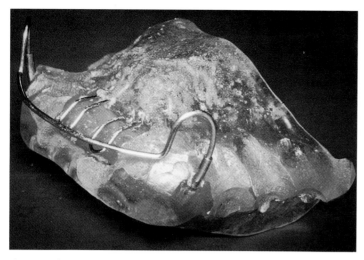

Fig. 6.8 The activator used for interceptive treatment of Class II division 2 malocclusion with a deep overbite.

becomes excessive. Due to the faulty incisor contact the mandible is guided backwards in closing from the rest position.

In the mixed dentition stage, such increased overbites are sometimes treated with an anterior bite plane. While this will be effective in reducing the incisal overbite, there are cogent arguments against using it at this stage of development. When a patient wears this appliance, overbite reduction is brought about by eruption of posterior teeth with additional deposition of alveolar bone in the molar region. At the stage in question, the deciduous molars will have almost or completely lost their eruption potential[11] and this means that the bite will be propped open on the first permanent molars. In the interests of stability the patient must continue to wear the appliance over a long period of time, perhaps even until the premolars and canines erupt and the occlusion of the incisors can be adjusted. Long-term wearing of removable appliances can give rise to serious problems of caries and soft tissue inflammation.

A better approach to these deep overbites in the mixed dentition is the activator or other

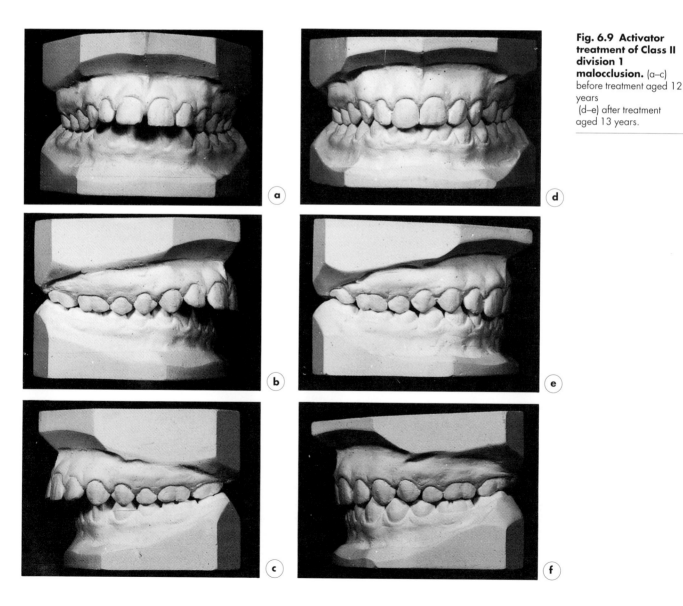

Fig. 6.9 Activator treatment of Class II division 1 malocclusion. (a–c) before treatment aged 12 years (d–e) after treatment aged 13 years.

functional appliance (Fig. 6.8). The activator used in this situation has springs for proclination of the upper incisors and the overbite may be reduced, partly by continued vertical development of the posterior dento-alveolar processes and partly due to forward growth of the mandible or mandibular dentition.

A great advantage is that the appliance need only be worn in the evenings and at night.

The general dental practitioner is well advised to refer posterior displacement cases and deep incisal overbites to an orthodontist.

Increased overjet

Many orthodontists leave the treatment of increased overjet on a skeletal I pattern until the canine and premolar teeth have erupted; others point out that proclined upper incisors may be more subject to trauma, especially if the lips are incompetent, and recommend early treatment in order to reduce the risk.[12] The use of the activator in relation to deep overbite has already been mentioned and this appliance is also useful in reducing an overjet during the mixed dentition stage. It will bring about retroclination of upper incisors, a favourable change in the buccal segment relationship and may allow mandibular growth to reach its full potential while limiting the forward growth of the maxilla.[13] The most favourable Class II division 1 cases for treatment with the activator have a post-normality amounting to half the breadth of a cusp and well-aligned upper and lower arches which are preferably spaced or at least not crowded (Fig. 6.9).

The effect of the activator in straightening the profile raises the possibility of treating a Class II malocclusion on a skeletal II pattern in two phases: a first interceptive phase with a functional appliance during the puberal growth spurt aimed at straightening the profile, and a second phase with fixed appliances to treat any crowding and align the teeth (Fig. 6.10).[14]

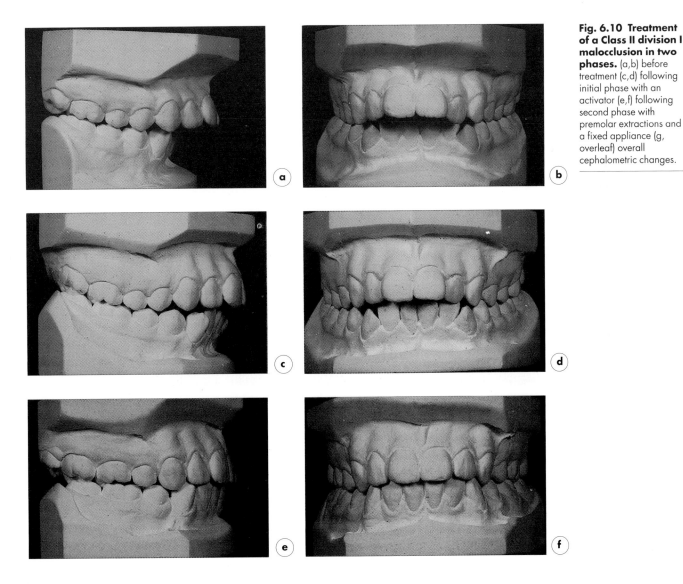

Fig. 6.10 Treatment of a Class II division I malocclusion in two phases. (a,b) before treatment (c,d) following initial phase with an activator (e,f) following second phase with premolar extractions and a fixed appliance (g, overleaf) overall cephalometric changes.

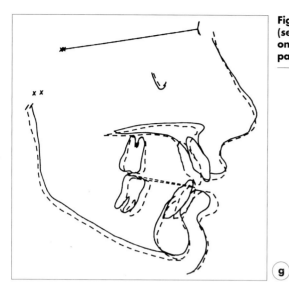

**Fig. 6.10g
(see caption
on previous
page).**

g

References

1 Thompson JR. The rest position of the mandible and its significance to dental science. *J Amer Dent Ass* 1946; **33**: 151–180.

2 Loh MK, Kerr WJS. The function regulator III: effects and indications for use. *Br J Orthod* 1985; **12**: 153–157.

3 Kerr WJS, Tenhave TR. A comparison of three appliance systems in the treatment of class III malocclusion. *Eur J Orthod* 1988; **10**: 203–214.

4 Thilander B. Chin-cap treatment for angle Class III malocclusion. *Eur Orthod Soc Trans* 1965: 311–327.

5 Adams C P, Richardson A. An assessment of the relationship of pre and post-eruptive lower incisor position to the facial pattern by serial cephalometric radiography. *Eur Orthod Soc Trans* 1967: 213– 223.

6 McMullan RE, Richardson A. Eruptive changes in the axial inclination of lower incisor teeth – a longitudinal study. *J Irish Dent Assoc* 1990; **36**: 53–56.

7 Allen RA, Connolly IH, Richardson A. Early treatment of class III incisor relationship using the chincap appliance. *Eur J Orthod* 1993; **15**: 371–376.

8 Abu Alhaija E, Richardson A. Long term effect of the chincap on hard and soft tissues. *Eur J Orthod* (in press).

9 Profitt WR, White RP. *Surgical orthodontic treatment.* St Louis: Mosby-Year Book Inc. 1991.

10 Leighton BC. The early development of cross-bites. *Trans Br Soc Study Orthod* 1966: 93–100.

11 Begg P R. *Orthodontic theory and technique.* Philadelphia: WB. Saunders, 1965 pp 48–49.

12 Burden DJ. An investigation of the association between overjet size, lip coverage, and traumatic injury to maxillary incisors. *Eur J Orthod* 1995; **17**: 513–517.

13 Trayfoot J, Richardson A. Angle Class II division 1 malocclusions treated by the Andresen method: an analysis of 17 cases. *Br Dent J* 1968; **124**: 516–519.

14 Richardson A, McCartney TI. Combined treatment methods in severe class II division 1 malocclusion with lower incisor crowding. *Am J Orthod* 1973; **63**: 581–587.

Summary of evidence for Chapter 6

Topic	Findings	Author/s
Mandibular rest position	Mandible assumes its positional relationship to the head by third month of life and thereafter does not change. Not affected by presence or absence of teeth. Normal free-way space 2–3mm. Bite may be raised in displacements with overclosure.	Thompson 1946[1]. Cephalometric x-rays in rest position of 75 children repeated after 8yrs, 16 having ortho treatment, 30 edentulous adults repeated after 4yrs.
Appliance systems in treatment of incisor Class III compared	Similar results for the 3 systems: Changes in mandibular posture, incisor inclinations, face height and SNB. FRIII associated with greatest change in skeletal relationships and change in cranial base angle.	Kerr & Tenhave 1988[3]. Conventional and tensor analysis of Class III incisor relation treated by FRIII, upper removable or Edgewise appliances.
Lower incisor inclinations	Lower incisors were always more proclined after eruption than before. The average difference was 13°.	Adams & Richardson 1967[5]. Longitudinal cephalometric study of 24F,26M between 5 and 11yrs.
Lower incisor inclinations	Greatest rate of proclination in first year after eruption. Diminution in proclination not related to occlusal contact.	McMullan & Richardson 1990[6]. Longitudinal cephalometric study of 18F,14M from 5–10yrs.
Effects of chincap with upper removable appliance	Short term: Proclination of upper and retroclination of lower incisors. No change in ANB or SNB. Mandible rotated clockwise. Long term: Overjet remained positive. Continued proclination of upper and retroclination of lower incisors. Mandible grew more in treated cases.	Alhaija & Richardson.[8] Longitudinal cephalometric study of 9F,14M Class IIIs treated with chincap and upper removable appliance. Review 1yr. after treatment. Matched controls.
Crossbites changes	High proportion of crossbites eliminated at changeover especially if associated with sucking habit and displacement.	Leighton 1966[10]. Longitudinal cast study of 19 crossbites from birth to permanent dentition.
Overjet and lip coverage as predictors of injury to upper incisors	15% had injuries. Sex differences in prevalence not significant. Overjet beyond 3.5mm and inadequate lip coverage increase risk. Lip coverage better predictor of injury than overjet.	Burden 1995[12]. 530F,577M age 11–12yrs in Northern Ireland examined for overjet, lip coverage and injury to upper incisors
Functional appliances (Andresen)	Retroclination of upper incisors. Significant differences in skeletal pattern.	Trayfoot & Richardson 1968[13]. Longitudinal study of 17 cases with matched controls.

7 Spacing and crowding

The evidence-based findings are summarised on pages 65 and 66.

Primary (innate) spacing or crowding of the teeth is caused by a faulty relationship between the triad of jaw size, arch perimeter and tooth size. The size of the jaw limits the relationship of the apices to one another, the arch perimeter limits the relationship of the crowns and the total mesio-distal crown size comes between the two.

Primary spacing

Some isolated spaces between teeth are caused by local factors such as absence of teeth, habits, unerupted supernumerary teeth, a prominent fraenum or loss of permanent teeth and will be dealt with in Chapter 8.

Generalised spacing between the teeth is uncommon in Caucasian subjects but common in patients of some other ethnic backgrounds. There seems little or no dental health detriment in generalised spacing and space closure with appliances is notoriously unstable. Patients with spaced dentitions who insist on space closure for cosmetic reasons usually have to accept permanent retention or creation of artificial tooth substance by the restorative dentist.

Primary crowding

Primary crowding may become manifest in the permanent dentition at age 7–9 years on eruption of the incisors, at 10–12 years on eruption of the canines, premolars and second molars or during the late teens in the form of late labial segment imbrication or impacted third molars. It is noteworthy that the earlier signs of crowding appear at the times of special vigilance listed in Chapter 2.

Early incisor crowding at 7–8 years

Early crowding may be apparent on eruption of the incisor teeth. The teeth are unable to escape from their crowded developmental positions so that the upper lateral incisors are usually trapped palatally between the centrals and deciduous canines, and the lower lateral incisors usually appear on the lingual side of the arch in rotated positions.

Mild crowding of incisors when they first erupt need not receive active treatment since a surprising amount of natural improvement may occur through spontaneous proclination, lateral jaw growth and encroachment on the leeway space following loss of the deciduous canines (Fig. 7.1). The decrease in crowding at this stage averages 0.9mm but may be as large as 4.48mm.[1]

Nonetheless, there may be a case for making maximum advantage of the leeway space in marginal incisor crowding. This raises the question of the size of the leeway space in a particular patient. In the average Caucasian subject, 21 or 22mm between the distal surface of the lateral incisor and the mesial surface of the first permanent molar will be sufficient to accommodate the canine and premolar teeth.

(a)   (b)

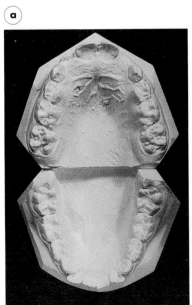
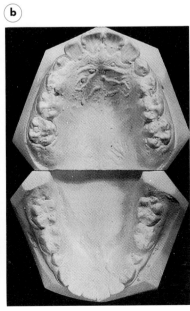

Fig. 7.1 (a) Lower incisor crowding at age 7.5 years.
(b) Spontaneous improvement by age 11 years.

Mixed dentition analysis

A more precise estimate of space requirements is the Holy Grail of interceptive orthodontists and is referred to as mixed dentition analysis. Almost all analyses depend to a greater or lesser extent on the good correlation which usually exists between the size of the lower incisors and the size of the unerupted canine and premolars.

Takana and Johnston[2] use the following equations:

Upper arch

The sum of the mesio-distal breadths of the canine and premolars in one quadrant = Half of the sum of the mesio-distal breadths of all the lower incisors + 11.0mm

Lower arch

The sum of the mesio-distal breadths of the canine and premolars in one quadrant = Half the sum of the mesio-distal breadths of all the lower incisors + 10.5mm

Moyers[3] presents a system in the form of probability tables. Having selected the sum of the mesio-distal breadths of lower incisors measured in a particular patient, the sum of the canine and premolar breadths can be read off directly. Similar data for Indian subjects are presented by Singh and Nanda .[4]

The accuracy of prediction can be improved by incorporating the sizes of the premolars measured on intra-oral films taken with a long cone technique. Data from Hixon and Oldfather,[5] revised by Staley and Kerber,[6] are shown graphically in Figure 7.2. This is generally held to be the most accurate of mixed dentition analyses. The mesio-distal breadths of the lower central and lateral incisors are added to the radiographic breadths of both premolars in the same quadrant. Entering this value on the graph allows the size of the unerupted canine and premolars to be predicted.

Space management

Utilisation of the leeway space to accommodate lower incisors can be done with a simple removable appliance having Adams clasps on the first molars or, more positively, with bands on the first permanent molars and a lingual arch in 1.0mm wire (Fig. 7.3). These appliances prevent mesial movement of the first permanent molars which normally encroaches on the leeway space.[7] It is important to balance the advantages of this treatment in terms of incisor crowding against the implications for the occlusion of the first molars. If the first molars are in a Class II relationship it may be better to allow the lower molar to drift forward into Class I occlusion and accept marginal lower incisor crowding. Alternatively, the upper first molar may be moved distally with a removable or fixed appliance.

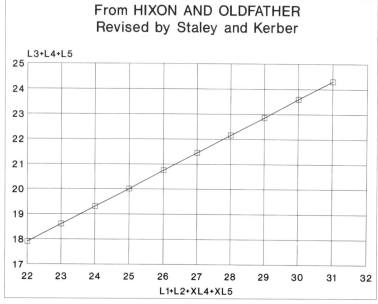

Fig. 7.2 Mixed dentition analysis.

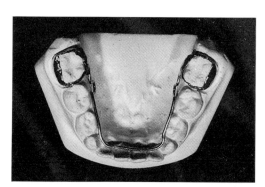

Fig. 7.3 Lingual arch.

This, in turn, will have implications for molar crowding which can be treated later by extraction of second molars. The best situation for leeway space utilisation is the lower arch with mild crowding of incisors amounting to less than 2mm and the first molars in Class I occlusion.

Expansion

It may be tempting to treat moderate degrees of crowding by increasing the arch perimeter, but the possibilities for this line of treatment are limited. Proclination of incisors should be reserved for upper incisors which are in a Class III relationship with the lowers. Rarely, lower incisors may be slightly proclined following reduction of a deep overbite or cessation of a thumb-sucking habit. Increasing the arch perimeter by lateral expansion was commonplace some years ago but the technique fell into abeyance for reasons neatly described as 'The Comedy of Expansion and the Tragedy of Relapse'.[8] British orthodontists subsequently became very cautious about arch expansion which came to be used not so much in the treatment of crowding, but in cases where upper molars were moved distally and must also be moved slightly buccally to correspond with a wider part of the lower arch, of unilateral crossbites with displacements and of cleft palate where permanent retention was planned in the form of bridge-work or a partial denture. Those

who are dedicated to expansion will over-expand to allow for some relapse.

In response to criticisms, justified or unjustified, that the treatment of crowding by extraction of premolar teeth leads to a concave profile, there has been a recent trend towards expansion of arches antero-posteriorly and laterally without extractions. This trend has received some encouragement from the commercial availability of preformed arches specifically for this purpose. The argument is that early expansion, when the dentition is actively developing, gives a better prospect of success than expansion at a later stage. It is too early to assess the validity of these arguments, most especially when patients treated in this way often wear bonded retainers, which will support the teeth in almost any position, or have proximal stripping which is a finely tuned reduction of tooth size. Bonded retainers carry the risk of decalcification, sometimes associated with undetected detachment of part of the retainer, and proximal stripping must have implications for the blood supply to the interdental papilla. By and large, this form of treatment is best avoided by the general practitioner.

Extraction

By far the most malleable determinant of crowding is tooth size, which may be conveniently reduced by extraction. In the context of

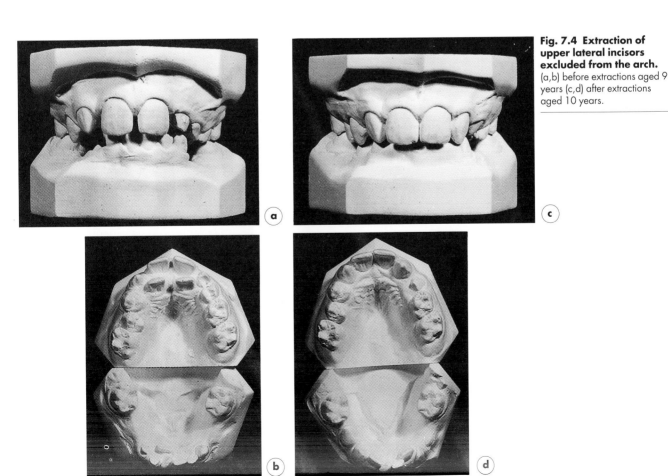

Fig. 7.4 Extraction of upper lateral incisors excluded from the arch. (a,b) before extractions aged 9 years (c,d) after extractions aged 10 years.

interceptive orthodontics, it is argued that if spaces are created in the right places and at the appropriate time, the adjacent teeth will grow into these spaces producing well-aligned arches with good approximal contacts and occlusion.

Very occasionally, extraction of an incisor tooth may give a good result (Fig. 7.4). It may be appropriate where the jaws are narrow and the teeth fanned out laterally, where the incisor is the seat of pathology such as dilaceration, dens in dente or pulp death or where the tooth is completely excluded from the arch. In the lower arch, the breadth between the canine teeth will diminish following extraction of an incisor. If there is a normal relationship between the sizes of the upper and lower teeth, extraction of a lower incisor compensated by extraction of upper premolars must lead to an abnormal overjet or an abnormal relationship in the buccal segments. Following extraction of an upper incisor, the distance between the canine teeth will become smaller but this will be more the result of drifting round the arch than narrowing of the arch in the canine region.

There are two well-recognised extraction therapies in the interceptive treatment of crowding. The first is serial extraction, introduced by Bunon in 1743,[9] described by Hotz,[10] popularised by Kjellgren,[11] and examined more critically by Dewel.[12] The second is extraction of first permanent molars strongly advocated by Wilkinson,[13,14] and by John Hunter and Joseph Fox as far back as the 18th century.[15,16]

Serial extraction

The three steps in a serial extraction are:

- When the lateral incisors are erupting in crowded positions, all four deciduous canines are removed to allow spontaneous alignment of the laterals. This very early loss of deciduous canines may also delay eruption of the permanent canines which is favourable in serial extraction.
- When the roots of the first deciduous molars are half resorbed, they are removed in order to promote early eruption of first premolars.
- When the first premolars are in the early stages of eruption, they are removed to make way for the erupting canines. It is important to extract first premolars on both sides at the same time in order to preserve the midline.

Serial extraction is not applicable in every patient where the erupting permanent incisors are crowded. The indications are usually listed as:

- The child should be aged 8–9 years and the incisors substantially crowded.
- The fundamental arch relationship should be Angle Class I.
- The overbite should be normal or reduced.

All the permanent teeth should be present in good positions.
- The first permanent molars should have a good prognosis.
- The first premolars should be closer to eruption than the canines.

Serial extraction should be avoided in skeletal II or skeletal III jaw relationships, where the face is unduly long or short, where a tight lower lip would retrocline lower incisors, or where the facial profile is substantially concave as judged by the position of the lower incisors to the A-Po line and the lips to the E line.

It is rather rare to find a patient who fulfils all of the serial extraction criteria to the letter. How much latitude should be allowed calls for clinical judgement and a consultant opinion. It is important to avoid complicating any subsequent orthodontic treatment by allowing overmuch space closure or deepening of the overbite which tends to occur in serial extraction cases.[17]

Most of the spontaneous proclination of lower incisors while they are actively erupting, occurs during the first post-eruptive year.[18] Since this rounding out process will make some space for crowded incisors, it is best to delay decisions on serial extraction until at least a year after the incisor teeth first appear in the mouth.

It would be normal to find the first premolar developmentally ahead of the canine in the upper arch but the opposite in the lower.[19] This eruption order in the lower arch may give rise to difficulties when the canine erupts early in a crowded position and the unerupted first premolar cannot be readily extracted. Some orthodontists advocate surgical enucleation of first premolars in these cases, but most take the view that such surgical trauma is not justified in circumstances which can be met by premolar extraction and appliance therapy at a later stage. In theory, the incisors, canines and second premolars should erupt in good alignment following the serial extraction procedure. In practice, however, careful monitoring is needed and a space maintainer sometimes required to hold open spaces for the upper canines. Most patients having serial extractions benefit from some subsequent appliance therapy which will be shorter and simpler than if crowding had been allowed to develop before orthodontic intervention.[11] There is no significant difference in irregularity, 10 years out of retention, between cases treated by serial extractions followed by appliance therapy and those treated by first premolar extractions and appliance therapy in the permanent dentition.[20] Figure 7.5 shows a good result following serial extractions without appliance therapy. Guidelines for serial extractions are available on computer disk from the author*.

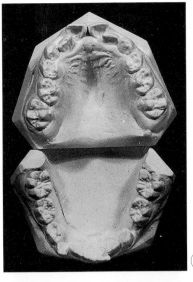
(a)

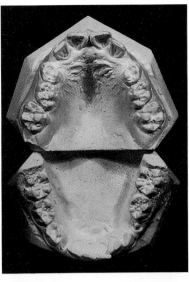
(c)

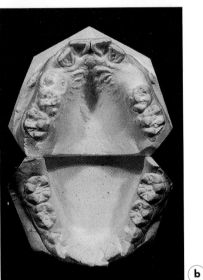
(b)

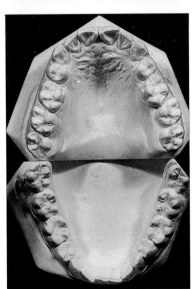
(d)

Fig. 7.5 (a) Crowding of lateral incisors at age 8 years: the deciduous canines were extracted. (b) one year later: the positions of the lateral incisors have improved; the first deciduous molars were extracted (c) one year later: the first premolars were extracted as they erupted (d) tooth positions at age 19 years: the third molars have erupted.

Elective extraction of first permanent molars

Extraction of all four first permanent molars seems to give the best results in the following circumstances:

- The child should be aged 8–9 years and have some evidence of crowding.
- The fundamental arch relationship should be normal (Angle Class I).
- The skeletal pattern should be Class I.
- The overbite should be normal or reduced.
- All the permanent teeth should be present.
- The first molars should be carious.
- The unerupted lower second premolar should not be distally inclined, spaced from the first premolar or outside the control of the second deciduous molar roots.

Similarities between the indications for first molar extractions and serial extractions will be obvious. The major differences lie in the prognosis for the first molars and the fact that serial extractions yield more space for relief of incisor crowding. First molar extractions, on the other hand, give more space for eruption of crowded second premolars and second and third molars.

The reasons and evidence supporting the selection criteria for extraction of all four first molars are as follows:

Age 8–9 years: Although 8–9 years of age is usually given as the optimum time for first molar extractions, the chronological age is not as important as the stage of dental maturity, with particular reference to the development of the lower second molar. If a lower first molar is extracted after eruption of the second molar the second molar tips mesially leading to poor approximal contacts.[21–23] More satisfactory space closure, angulations and approximal contacts are produced in the lower arch if the first molar is extracted before eruption of the second molar.[23] Timing is not so important in the upper arch where a second molar will move forward satisfactorily after eruption.

Angle Class I arch relationship: Since an approximately equal amount of tooth substance is removed from upper and lower arches, the best occlusion is achieved when the pre-existing occlusion is Class I. A slight reduction in overjet occurs in Class I cases but there is no overjet reduction in Class II division 1 cases.[24]

Class I skeletal pattern: Longitudinal studies, some of them extending to 25 years after the extractions, have shown that the most favourable outcomes were in skeletal I cases.[21] Prophylactic extraction of all first molars should be avoided in skeletal II or skeletal III jaw relationships and where the face is unduly short.

Normal or reduced overbite: This is a traditional criterion based on clinical opinion. The evidence is that the effects on overbite are not as great as was once believed, providing the skeletal pattern is Class I (Fig. 7.6).[24,25]

Presence of all permanent teeth: This criterion applies particularly to second premolars which are frequently absent. It cannot apply to third molars because many have not developed at age 8–9 years.

The first molars should be carious: Extraction of first permanent molars is rarely the orthodontic treatment of choice. Most orthodontists need caries in first permanent molars and a poor prognosis before they can be persuaded that first molars should be removed. One prominent orthodontist has stated that extraction of first molars as against premolars

doubles the orthodontic treatment time and halves the prognosis.[26]

Unerupted lower second premolar: Unerupted lower second premolars are frequently distally inclined and will continue to erupt distally following removal of the first molar (Fig. 7.7).[23]

In summary, if the listed criteria are fulfilled, the results of extraction of all 4 first permanent molars may be acceptable (Fig. 7.8), but it is not a treatment that should be undertaken lightly and it is not the panacea that Wilkinson described.[13,14]

Enforced extraction of first permanent molars

Another aspect of first molar extractions is the situation where one first molar is sufficiently carious to warrant extraction. The questions facing the practitioner relate to the most favourable age or dental stage for the extraction (assuming he has some choice) and whether he should compensate for the extraction by removing the opposing first molar (a compensating extraction), the first molar on the other side of the same arch (a balancing extraction), or all 4 first molars. Against the background of conflicting evidence in a complicated situation many practitioners, with some justification, limit themselves to treating the immediate pathological condition. There are 196 combinations of variables to be considered, not all of which can be covered in this book. Practitioners can spare themselves strenuous mental activity by using computer

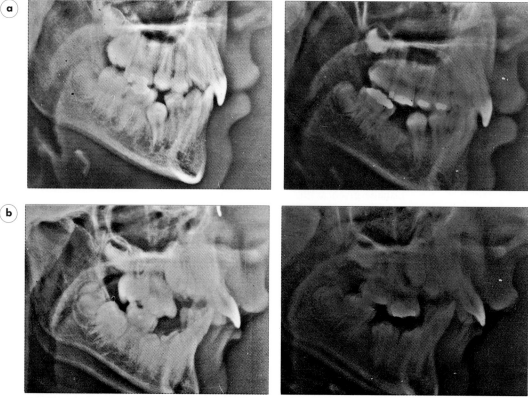

Fig. 7.6 Increase in overbite and overjet following extraction of lower first permanent molars (a) in Class I incisor relationship (b) in Class II division 1 incisor relationship.

programs, one of which is available from the author**.

The general guidelines which follow assume that the practitioner has some choice in the timing of extractions and that root treatment may be a viable option in some cases:

- A lower first molar should be extracted before eruption of the second molar.
- Extraction of a lower first molar should be delayed if the lower second premolar is distally inclined.

- A removable appliance with an anterior bite plane or a functional appliance should be provided before or shortly after extracting a lower first molar in skeletal class II cases or where the overjet or overbite is increased.
- Extraction of an upper first molar should be delayed until the second molar erupts when it is intended that the extraction space be used to treat an increased overjet or crowded upper incisors.
- All teeth should be present.

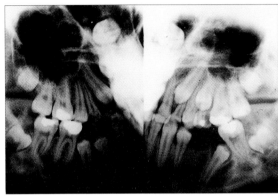

Fig. 7.7 Extraction of the lower left first molar has allowed the second premolar to tip distally and become impacted against the second molar.

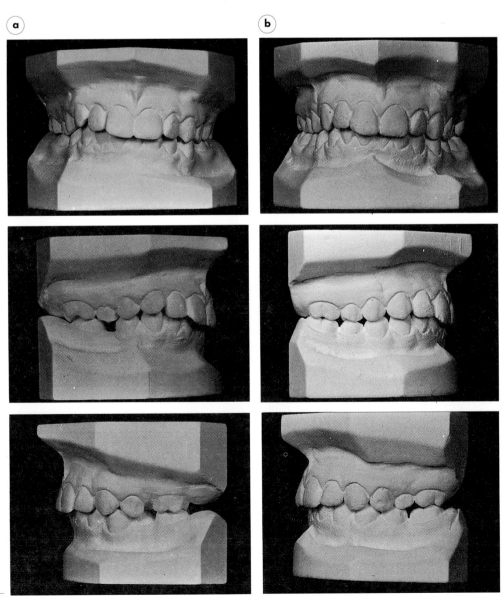

Fig. 7.8 Tooth positions before and after extraction of the first permanent molars. (a) before (b) after.

- If a lower first molar must be extracted, the opposing first molar should be extracted in mildly crowded Class I cases.
- If an upper first molar must be extracted, compensating extraction of the opposing lower first molar is not indicated.
- Balancing extractions to preserve the midline are not indicated unless the teeth are extracted at a very early age.

The rationale behind these guidelines is as follows:

Early extraction of lower first molars and second molar positions: Late extraction of a lower first molar after second molar eruption leads to much mesial tipping and rolling of the second molar (unless much of the extraction space can be taken up by a crowded second premolar). This faulty position of the second molar is one of the major points of criticism of first molar extraction results. On the other hand, extraction of the first molar before eruption and root formation of the second molar is followed by intraosseous mesial movement of the second molar and much more satisfactory occlusal and approximal relationships after eruption.[22,23,27]

Late extraction of first molars and second premolar positions: The lower second premolar is often distally inclined at an early stage of development. During normal eruption it is guided occlusally by the distal root of the deciduous molar or, failing this, by the mesial surface of the first permanent molar. If the first molar is removed at an early stage, there is a tendency for the second premolar to erupt distally and become impacted against the second molar or to leave a space between the first and second premolars (see Fig. 7.7).[23,28]

Appliance therapy in cases of increased overbite or overjet: Extraction of lower first molars may be followed by a substantial increase in the overbite and overjet if the pre-existing overbite and overjet are increased and the incisors are proclined. This may be partly due to retroclination of lower incisors and partly to counter-clockwise rotation of the mandible.[29]

Utilisation of upper first molar spaces: space created by extraction of an upper first molar is taken up rapidly by mesial movement of the second molar with no possibility of controlling it while it is still unerupted. If much space is needed to treat upper incisor crowding or an increased overjet, it is wise to fit an upper appliance to control the second molar before the extraction. However, it is worth keeping in mind that space is lost in transferring an upper first molar space to the front of the mouth with appliances. If there is gross crowding or a large overjet and the third molar is well-formed, a more practical proposition may be extraction of the first molar to allow mesial movement of the second molar and eruption of the third molar followed later by bilateral extraction of premolars and appliance therapy.

Presence of all teeth: The presence of all teeth (with the possible exception of third molars) should be ascertained radiographically before balancing or compensating extractions are carried out. The unerupted teeth should be in favourable positions and free from developmental defects.

Compensatory upper extraction: In most cases, an upper first molar will over-erupt following extraction of the lower antagonist.[30] This leads to premature contacts and impaired closure of the lower extraction space because the lower second molar becomes snagged behind the over-erupted upper first molar. Extraction of lower first molars is usually compensated by extraction of the corresponding upper molar but not necessarily at the same time.

No compensatory lower extractions: The tendency for lower first molars to over-erupt after loss of their antagonists is much less than in the upper. Compensatory extraction of lower first molars may bring more detriment than benefit in terms of residual spacing and poor approximal contacts and angulations.[22]

Midlines: First molars are sufficiently distally placed that movement of the midline following extraction of a first molar is rarely a problem.[31,32] Compensating extractions on the other side of the mouth are usually not essential.

Crowding in the buccal segments

The age for special vigilance of buccal segment crowding is 10–12 years when the canine, premolar and second molar teeth are erupting. If the dentist is seeing the patient for the first time at this stage, it is best to undertake a complete review of the space conditions. Where the jaws are narrow and the canine teeth buccally inclined or where the canines are distally inclined, there may be an argument in favour of extracting a lateral incisor if it is the seat of pathology or excluded from the arch (Fig. 7.9). The midline will move to the side of the extraction if has not already done so.

In situations where the canine is mesially inclined, such as jaws which are short anteroposteriorly, or where the buccal segments have drifted forwards, extraction of a tooth distal to the canine is best. In the absence of gross decay influencing the choice of teeth for extraction, removal of first premolars is usually indicated if the crowding is to be treated interceptively. These teeth are strategically placed for the treatment of incisor, canine and premolar crowding and their early eruption in the upper arch makes them accessible for extraction before the neighbouring teeth erupt. Interceptive extraction of

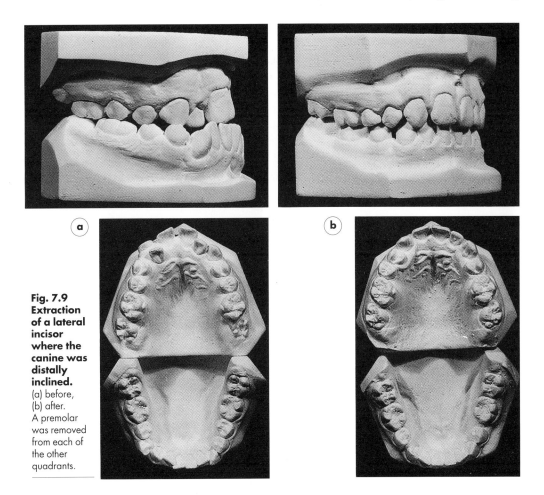

**Fig. 7.9
Extraction
of a lateral
incisor
where the
canine was
distally
inclined.**
(a) before,
(b) after.
A premolar
was removed
from each of
the other
quadrants.

first premolars should be done at the time the canines are in their active eruption phase. Especially in the lower arch, the canines will drift distally into the extraction sites of their own accord, giving relief from the incisor crowding (Fig. 7.10).

Skilful judgement is required in deciding which patients can safely be left to improve spontaneously. Space created by the extraction of first premolars will close partly by distal movement of canines and partly by mesial movement of the second premolars and the teeth behind them. The danger is that mesial drift of the posterior teeth will occupy too much of the extraction space, leaving insufficient space for the incisors and canine. If there seems any possibility of this happening, an orthodontic opinion should be sought before any treatment decision is made. Finally, if there is still some doubt, a space maintainer in the shape of a lingual arch or removable appliance may be fitted.

Although extraction of first premolars which is not followed by appliance therapy is frequently denigrated by the term 'drifto-dontics', the evidence is that the extraction spaces usually close completely,[33] that spon-taneous uprighting of the canine and second premolar occurs after the space has closed[34] and that 20 years after the extraction it is difficult to distinguish between those patients who wore appliances and those who did not.[35]

In rare cases, extraction of a hypoplastic or grossly displaced canine may give an acceptable result (Fig. 7.11). The disadvantages of extracting canines are a slight accentuation of the naso-labial fold or, more importantly, an unsightly mesio-labial rotation of the upper first premolar so that the palatal cusp becomes obvious.

Where there is secondary crowding following premature loss of a second deciduous molar, the second premolar is frequently excluded from the arch on the lingual or palatal side. Extraction of the second premolar is often a very satisfactory answer to this problem especially if the canine and first premolar have erupted early into good positions.

In terms of the interceptive treatment of primary crowding, there still remains the problem of crowding in the molar region. In the lower arch, this usually takes the form of impacted third molars or even second molars, whereas in the upper jaw the crowding is usually

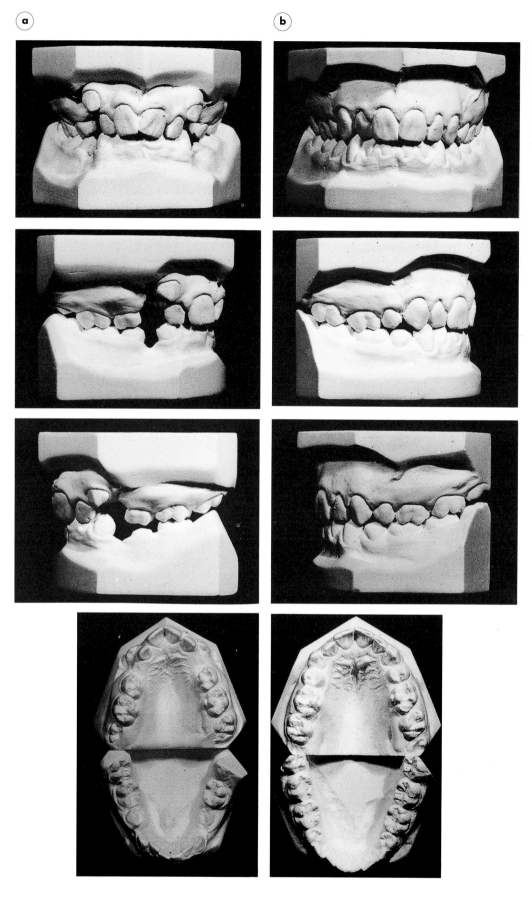

Fig. 7.10 Spontaneous alignment of canines following extraction of first premolars at age 10 years. (a) shortly after extractions (b) aged 16 years. The only appliance worn was an upper space maintainer.

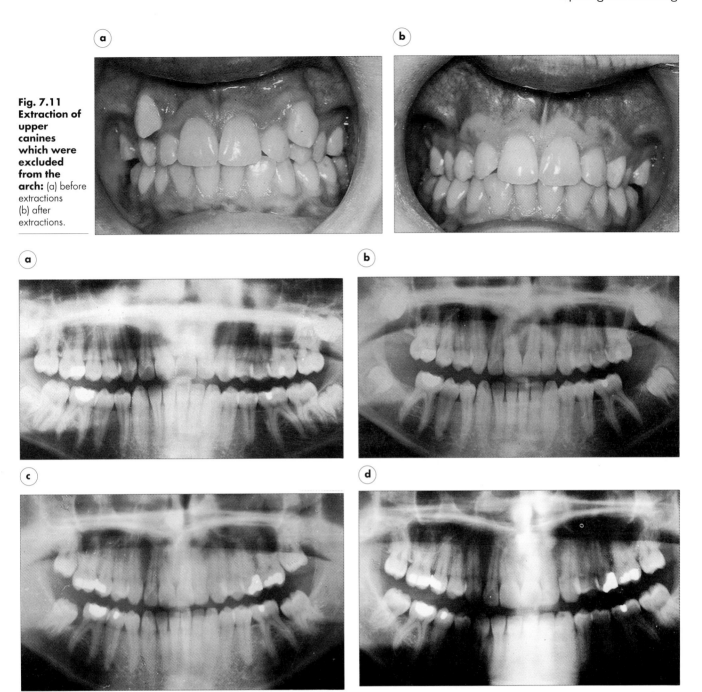

Fig. 7.11 Extraction of upper canines which were excluded from the arch: (a) before extractions (b) after extractions.

Fig. 7.12 Eruption of third molars after extraction of second molars: (a) aged 13 years (b) aged 14 years (c) aged 15 years (d) aged 16 years.

recognisable by stepping or stacking of the molar teeth. Removal of the third molars may solve the problem and indeed there are the possibilities of interceptive surgical approaches such as germectomy or lateral trepanation.[36] These surgical approaches do involve the patient in procedures greater than simple forceps extraction and it is appropriate to consider the simple extraction of teeth anterior to the third molar as treatment of this form of crowding.

Extraction of second molars

The following guidelines for extraction of lower second molars to reduce impaction of third molars have been proposed:[37,38]

- When the crown of the third molar is

completely formed but root formation has not started.
- When the third molar is in a mesio-angular position making an angle of less than 30 degrees to the long axis of the first molar or where the occlusal surface makes an angle of between 20 and 60 degrees to the occlusal plane of the erupted molar and premolars.

Extraction of second molars at about this stage seems to permit eruption of third molars in good alignment in the majority of cases (Fig. 7.12). Subsequent work has shown that the timing of second molar extractions and the developmental stage and position of the third molars may not be as critical as the guidelines would imply.[39]

Following early removal of lower second molars, there is an average distal movement of lower first molars and a slight decrease in crowding of the more anterior teeth.[40] In a non-extraction control group there was, on average, mesial movement of lower first molars and increasing crowding in the anterior part of the arch. Extraction of second molars may also allow spontaneous eruption of crowded second premolars into good alignment if they are not far from the line of the arch. It is worth remembering, however, that extraction of a lower second molar may allow over-eruption of the upper second molar leading to faulty occlusal contacts so that extraction of all four second molars is a better treatment than extraction of lower second molars alone.

Secondary crowding

Secondary crowding is frequently caused by extraction of deciduous teeth. Early loss of deciduous incisors in spaced arches may have remarkably little effect on crowding. Removal of a deciduous molar, however, usually produces a variably extensive collapse of the buccal segment so that there is insufficient space for the succedaneous teeth. Most important of all is loss of the second deciduous molar because the first permanent molar comes forward very readily.

The pattern of space closure following extraction of a deciduous molar is typically rapid in the first few months, with the rate of closure diminishing thereafter. In one study[41] an average of 1.37mm, 0.86mm, 0.77mm and 0.59mm were lost during the first 4 periods of 6 months after deciduous molar extraction. Spaces close more rapidly in the upper arch than in the lower and spaces close more quickly following loss of a second, than of a first deciduous molar. In some cases, spaces close almost entirely by mesial movement of posterior teeth, in some cases by distal movement of anterior teeth, but in the majority by a combination of these movements in varying degrees.[41]

Space maintenance

While the best treatment of premature extraction is true prevention so that the need for extraction does not arise, the interceptive orthodontist may still control space closure following unavoidable extraction by the use of a space maintainer. In view of the high rate of space closure which occurs immediately after the extraction is carried out, it is imperative that the space maintainer is inserted immediately after the tooth is extracted. Space maintainers may be fixed or removable (Fig. 7.13).

Although the design of space maintainers may be simple, deciding where to use them is more complex. In this regard, patients fall into four categories:

- Where the arches are generous in size or where there is hypodontia, there is no need to maintain space because space closure will be desirable (Fig. 7.14a).
- In cases where there is some crowding of the anterior teeth amounting to appreciably less than the breadth of a premolar in each quadrant, there is no need to maintain space because extraction of premolars or molars will be part of the treatment (Fig. 7.14b).
- Between these first two categories there is the condition where there will be just enough space to accommodate the teeth in acceptable alignment. This is the classical indication for using a space maintainer (Fig. 7.14c).
- The last type of case is where extraction of a permanent tooth from the quadrant will give just enough space to accommodate the other teeth in good alignment. This degree of crowding is uncommon but space maintenance in these cases is essential.

A computer programme on the use of space maintainers is available from the author***.

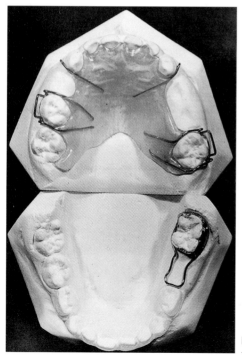

Fig. 7.13 Space maintainers.

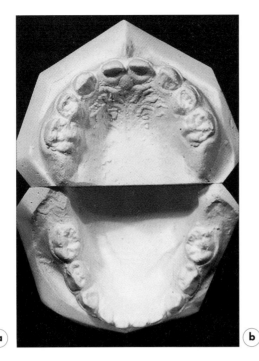
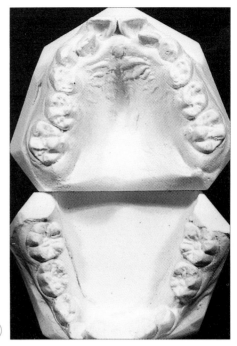
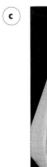
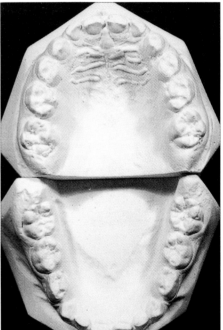

Fig. 7.14 (a) Spaced arches with absence of deciduous and permanent lateral incisors. Space maintenance would not be required following loss of a deciduous molar. **(b) Crowded arches:** extraction of permanent teeth will be necessary to treat the crowding; space maintenance would not be required following loss of a deciduous molar. **(c) Developing ideal occlusion:** space maintenance would be required following loss of a deciduous molar.

Late labial segment imbrication

This occurs between the ages of 13 and 18 years and may continue into adult life (Fig. 7.15). The aetiology is enigmatic and multifactorial. Some of the causes are given in Chapter 2.

In terms of treatment, extraction of second molars seems to be an effective interceptive manoeuvre.[39] Mild degrees of crowding are probably best accepted, while severe degrees may call for extractions and mechanical orthodontic treatment or re-treatment. The 'conservative' approach of stripping enamel from the approximal surfaces of the incisors is fashionable but many clinicians have concern about the possibility of a diminution in the blood supply to the approximal gingivae.

---

* Guidelines on serial extractions computed by Andrew Richardson and Terry Gregg
** Guidelines on extraction of first permanent molars computed by Andrew Richardson and Terry Gregg
*** Guidelines on space maintenance computed by Andrew Richardson and Terry Gregg

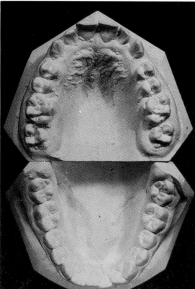

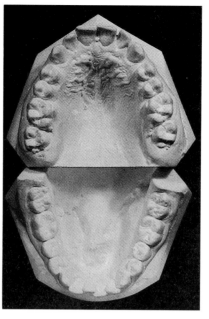

Fig. 7.15 Late labial segment imbrication (a) age 12.5 years, (b) age 15.5 years.

References

1 Lundy HJ, Richardson ME. Developmental changes in alignment of the lower labial segment. *Br J Orthod* 1995; **22**: 339–345.

2 Takana MM, Johnston LE. The prediction of the size of unerupted canines and premolars in a contemporary orthodontic population. *J Amer Dent Assoc* 1974; **88**: 798–801.

3 Moyers RE et al. *Standards of human occlusal development* Monograph 5, Craniofacial Growth Series, Ann Arbor, Michigan. University of Michigan 1976.

4 Singh M, Nanda RS. Prediction of tooth size and its clinical application. *J Indian Dent Assoc* 1972; **44**: 95–98.

5 Hixon EH, Oldfather RE. Estimation of the sizes of unerupted cusbid and bicusbid teeth. *Angle Orthod* 1958; **28**: 236–240.

6 Staley RN, Kerber RE. A revision of the Hixon and Oldfather mixed dentition prediction method. *Am J Orthod* 1980; **78**: 296–302.

7 Gianelly AA. Crowding: timing of treatment. *Angle Orthod* 1994; **64**: 415–418.

8 Townend BR. The comedy of expansion and the tragedy of relapse. *Dent Mag Oral Topics* 1956; **72**: 153–166.

9 Bunon R. *Essay sur les maladies des dents Briasson*: Paris 1743.

10 Hotz R. Active supervision of the eruption of the teeth by extraction. *Eur Orthod Soc Trans* 1947: 134–160.

11 Kjellgren B. Serial extraction as a corrective procedure in dental orthopaedic therapy. *Eur Orthod Soc Trans* 1948; 134–160.

12 Dewel BF. A critical analysis of serial extraction in orthodontic treatment. *Am J Orthod* 1959; **45**: 424–455.

13 Wilkinson AA. The first permanent molar again. *Br Dent J* 1940; **69**: 269–284.

14 Wilkinson AA. Early extraction of the first permanent molar as the best method of preserving the dentition as a whole. *Dent Record* 1944; **64**: 25–35, 51–58.

15 Hunter J. *The natural history of the human teeth*. 2nd ed. London, J Johnston 1778 p.81.

16 Fox J. *The natural history of the human teeth*. London, Thos Cox 1803 pp.63–64.

17 Ringenberg QM. Influence of serial extraction on growth and development of the maxilla and mandible. *Am J Orthod* 1967; **53**: 19–26.

18 McMullan RE, Richardson A. Eruptive changes in the axial inclination of lower incisors – A longitudinal study. *J Irish Dent Assoc* 1990; **36**: 53–56.

19 Kochhar R, Richardson A. The chronology and sequence of eruption of human permanent teeth in Northern Ireland. *Int J Paed Dent* 1998; **8**: 243–252.

20 Little RM, Riedel RA, Engst DE. Serial extraction of first premolars – postretention evaluation of stability and relapse. *Angle Orthod* 1990; **60**: 255–262.

21 Thunold K. Early loss of the first molars –25 years after. *Eur Orthod Soc Trans* 1970: 349–365.

22 Plint DA. The effect on the occlusion of the loss of one or more first permanent molars – with special reference to the third permanent molars. *Eur Orthod Soc Trans* 1970: 329–336.

23 Hallett GEM, Burke P. Symmetrical extraction of first permanent molars. Factors controlling results in the lower arch. *Eur Orthod Soc Trans* 1961: 238–255.

24 McEwen JD, McHugh WD. An epidemiological investigation into the effects of the loss of first permanent molar teeth. *Eur Orthod Soc Trans* 1970: 337–348.

25 Mc Ewen JD, McHugh WD, Hitchin AD. The effects of extraction of the four first permanent molars. *Eur Orthod Soc Trans* 1964: 344–356.

26 Mills JRE. *Principles and practice of Orthodontics*. 2nd.ed. Edinburgh, Churchill Livingstone, 1987. p.123.

27 Thilander B, Skagius S. Orthodontic sequelae of extraction of permanent first molars – a longitudinal study. *Eur Orthod Soc Trans* 1970: 429–442.

28 Dahan J. A gnatho-odontometric analysis of cases with extraction of the first permanent molars. *Eur Orthod Soc Trans* 1970: 367-381.

29 Richardson A. Spontaneous changes in the incisor relationship following extraction of lower first permanent molars. *Br J Orthod* 1979; **6**: 85–90.

30 Enunlu N. An investigation into the effects of early extraction of first permanent molars on alveolar processes and jaw bones. *Eur Orthod Soc Trans* 1971: 439–450.

31 Salzman JA. Rate and direction of orthodontic change and effect on the incidence of caries in five hundred adolescents following caries, filling or extraction of the first permanent molars. *J Amer Dent Assoc* 1939; **26**: 1991–2001.

32 Salzman JA. Variation in tooth position following extraction of first molars in relation to incidence and distribution of caries. *J Dent Res* 1940; **19**: 17–33.

33 Cookson AM. Space closure following the loss of lower first premolars. *Trans Brit Soc Study Orthod* 1970: 27–32.

34 Swessi DM, Stephens CD. The spontaneous effects of lower first premolar extraction on the mesio-distal angulation of adjacent teeth and the relationship of this to extraction space closure in the long term. *Eur J Orthod* 1993; **15**: 503–511.

35 Persson M, Persson E, Skagius S. Long-term spontaneous changes following removal of all first premolars in Class I cases with crowding. *Eur J Orthod* 1989; **11**: 271–282.

36 Henry CB. Excision of the developing mandibular third molar by lateral trepanation. *Br Dent J* 1969; **127**: 111–118.

37 Cryer BS. Third molar eruption and the effect of extraction of adjacent teeth. *Dent Practit* 1967; **17**: 405–416.

38 Huggins DG, McBride LJ. The eruption of lower third molars following the loss of lower second molars: a longitudinal cephalometric study. *Br J Orthod* 1978; **5**: 13–20.

39 Richardson ME, Richardson A. Lower third molar development subsequent to second molar extraction. *Am J Orthod Dentofac Orthop* 1993; **104**: 566–574.

40 Richardson ME, Mills K. Late lower arch crowding the effect of second molar extraction. *Am J Orthod Dentofac Orthop* 1990; **98**: 242–246.

41 Richardson ME. The relationship between the relative amount of space present in the deciduous dental arch and the rate and degree of space closure subsequent to the extraction of a deciduous molar. *Trans Brit Soc Study Orthod* 1965: 51–58.

Summary of evidence for Chapter 7

Topic	Findings	Author/s
Labial segment crowding	Decrease in crowding of lower incisors between their eruption and eruption of canines. Increase during 3 years following eruption of second molars.	Lundy & Richardson ME 1995.[1] Longitudinal cast and cephalometric study of 28F,20M from eruption of lower incisors to 3yrs after eruption of second molars.
Mixed dentition analysis	Correlation coefficients between sum lower incisors and canine+ premolars were 0.625 in upper and 0.648 in lower. Prediction equation in text.	Takana & Johnston 1974.[2] Casts of 506 subjects of European ancestry.
Mixed dentition analysis	Probability charts based on good correlation between widths of mandibular incisors and unerupted canines and premolars.	Moyers et al. 1976.[3] Dental cast study of large number of North American white children.
Mixed dentition analysis	Sum of mesio-distal widths of lower incisors strongly correlated with mesio-distal widths of canines and premolars.	Singh & Nanda 1972.[4] Dental cast study of 104 Indian children.
Mixed dentition analysis	(1+2) + (4+5) Predicted 3+4+5 23mm 18.4mm 24 19.0 25 19.7 26 20.3 27 21.0 28 21.6 29 22.3 30 22.9	Hixon & Oldfather 1958.[5] Cast (1+2) and radiograph (4+5) measurements of 41 subjects compared with 3+4+5 after eruption.
Serial extraction	On average there was a deeper overbite in serial extraction groups due to lingual tipping of incisors. No differences in soft tissue profile. Active treatment time reduced from 19 months to 12.7 months in serial extraction cases.	Ringenberg 1967.[17] Six cephalometric studies of more than 200 cases with controls are reported.
Lower incisor inclinations	Greatest rate of proclination in first year after eruption. Diminution in proclination not related to occlusal contact.	McMullan & Richardson 1990.[18] Longitudinal cephalometric study of 18F,14M from 5 to 10yrs.
Eruption ages and sequences	Results quoted refer to cases without premature loss. Females before males except for second molars. Lower before upper except for premolars. No difference between sides. Premature loss of deciduous teeth delays age of eruption except upper premolars. Most common sequence of eruption unique to the subject.	Kochhar & Richardson 1998.[19] Longitudinal study of 276 children in Northern Ireland.
Serial extractions and appliance and later extractions and appliance compared.	All showed increasing irregularity after retention. No difference between serial extractions + appliance and later extractions + appliance but 12 months shorter treatment in serial extractions.	Little et al 1990.[20] 30 serial extraction + appl. compared with later extraction of 4/4 + appl. 10yrs out of retention.
Loss of one or more first molars	Good results in upper. Residual space and tipping in lower. Crowding is beneficial. Best age 8–10yrs. Distal occlusion, deep bite and increased overjet are detrimental.	Thunold 1970.[21] Retrospective cast and X-ray study of 23F, 29M 25yrs after extraction.
Loss of one or more first molars	Majority of third molars erupted. Better axial inclinations of second molars, better contacts and less spacing in upper arch as against lower.	Plint 1970.[22] Retrospective cast and lateral x-ray study of 50F,25M.
Extraction of four first molars	Best results when lower teeth crowded. Results not related to tooth size. No significant change in overbite.	Hallett & Burke 1961.[23] Retrospective cast and mandibular X-rays of over 100 who had extraction of four first molars.
Loss of all first molars	Small increase in overbite. Significant overjet decrease in Class I no significant overjet change in other classes of malocclusion.	Mc Ewen & McHugh 1970.[24] Cross-sectional study of random sample 9,294 age 12yrs.
Loss of all first molars	Less anterior crowding and more anterior spacing in extraction cases. No significant difference in overbite but diminished overjet in extraction cases.	Mc Ewen et al. 1964.[25] Cross-sectional study of 481 who had lost all first molars and 1,198 who had not.
Loss of one or more first molars	Best stage for extraction: after eruption of laterals, before eruption of second molars. Crowding and presence of third molars favourable.	Thilander & Skagius 1970.[27] Longitudinal cast and 45° rotated cephalometric study of 103F,72M until spaces closed.

Topic (continued)	Findings	Author/s
Extraction of lower first molars	Overjet and overbite increased. Lower incisors retroclined, upper incisors proclined. Increase in overbite related to previous overbite and overjet and proclination of incisors.	Richardson 1979.[29] Longitudinal cephalometric study of 24F,19M before and 12 months after extraction of lower first molars.
Extraction of isolated first molars	Mesial drift in upper, distal drift of lower premolars. Over-eruption of opposing teeth.	Enunlu 1971.[30] Longitudinal cast study of 30 subjects.
Extraction of one or more first molars	Larger spaces open between premolars in lower arch following extraction. Elevation or continuous eruption of upper molar following loss of lower molar.	Salzman 1940.[32] Cross-sectional cast study of 500 who had lost one or more first molars and 1,440 who had not.
Spontaneous space closure following extraction of first premolars	Complete space closure in 83%. Acceptable alignment of incisors in 94 cases. Degree of closure related to total crowding. Presence of third molars not significant below 12 years.	Cookson 1970.[33] Longitudinal cast study of 118 subjects before and 5yrs after first premolar extractions.
Spontaneous space closure following extraction of first premolars	Maximum tipping 15 degrees. Greatest during first 6 months. Uprighting, especially of canine, in the long term. Excessive tipping exceptional.	Swessi & Stephens 1993.[34] Study casts of 8F,12M before extraction of lower first premolars, and at 13yrs after extraction.
Extraction of first premolars	Marked spontaneous arch alignment and space closure similar to treated sample. No detrimental effects on overbite or overjet. Lower incisor positions similar to normal occlusions. Tipping of teeth towards the extraction site not related to marginal bone height. Some late crowding in spite of extractions.	Persson et al. 1989.[35] Longitudinal clinical, cast and X-ray study of 21F,21M at age 30 who had extraction of all premolars at 10fiyrs 2 Control samples: normal occlusions and complete dentitions.
Extraction of lower second molars	Judged on final position of 8s and relief of crowding: 35% good, 40% fair, 25% poor. 70% good results if extraction at full crown formation of third molars and inclination of 8 not more than 30 degrees to long axis of 6.	Cryer 1967.[37] Longitudinal cast and radiograph study of 66 patients with extraction of one or both lower second molars.
Effect of lower second molar extraction on lower third molar eruption & post-eruption positions	All lower third molars erupted. 96% erupted in good positions assessed by scoring system.	Richardson ME & Richardson 1993.[39] Longitudinal cast and rotated cephalometric study of 63 treated by extraction of second molars.
Effect of second molar removal on crowding	Forward movement of first molars and increased crowding in non-extraction group. Distal movement of first molars and decreased crowding in extraction group.	Richardson ME. & Mills 1990.[40] Longitudinal cast & cephalometric study of 30 with second molar extractions and 30 without extractions.
Space closure after extraction of deciduous molars	More space lost in crowded arches. High correlations between space loss in first and subsequent 6 months. Most space lost in first 6 months. More rapid space closure in upper.	Richardson ME. 1965.[41] Longitudinal cast study of 30F,44M who had deciduous molars extracted.

8 Local irregularities

The evidence-based findings are summarised on pages 83 and 84.

Achieving a precise and watertight classification of local causes of malocclusion is notoriously difficult. Some items listed under local causes are malpositions or malocclusions in themselves and in some local irregularities there is more than one cause. Under the heading of local causes of malocclusion, Bennett[1] included factors which exert their influence principally in a single localised area of the mouth – sufficiently localised that they could be excluded from the heading of developmental defects of bone affecting a whole arch (such as crowding) and without affecting the relationship of the arches in any of the three planes of space. Of course, it is impossible to find an irregularity which is so precisely demarcated that it does not have any effect on adjacent and opposing teeth but, with these reservations, the local causes described by Bennett provide a convenient list of local problems which may serve to define the frontiers of this chapter. Having said that, it is interesting to note that patients having one local anomaly may have another local anomaly elsewhere in the mouth.[2] The aetiology of so-called local anomalies may not be as local as the name suggests.

In general, local problems become noticeable at an early stage of occlusal development and respond favourably to early detection and interceptive treatment.

Missing teeth (hypodontia)

Absence of deciduous teeth is quite rare, with a prevalence of less than 1%. When it does occur, the upper lateral incisor is the tooth most often affected. Current concepts of tooth development would suggest that if the deciduous tooth is absent, the permanent tooth should also be absent. Excluding third molars, the prevalence of missing teeth in the permanent dentition is 3.3%, with females more commonly affected.[3]

The permanent teeth most frequently missing in Europeans[4] are third molars, lower second premolars, upper lateral incisors and, less commonly, lower central incisors (Fig. 8.1). It has been suggested that hypodontia is an evolutionary trait and that Nature is omitting the last tooth in each series (i.e. molar, premolar, incisor) to compensate for the evolutionary shortening of the jaws. This hypothesis rather falls down in relation to the lower central incisors but it is possible that absence of these teeth has a different aetiology.

Absence of many teeth (oligodontia) may be associated with delayed eruption, microdontia and an abnormal crown form of those teeth which are present. There may be other ectodermal defects such as sparse hair and deficient sweat glands. The dentition in these cases calls for the combined care of orthodontic and restorative specialists.

Absence of a few teeth is often symmetrical about the mid-line or there may be absence of the tooth on one side and microdontia of the corresponding tooth on the opposite side (Fig. 8.2).

In general, problems created by absence of a

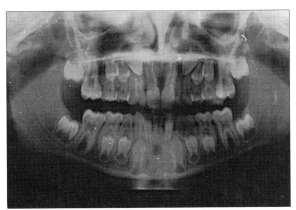

Fig. 8.1 Pantomogram showing absence of upper permanent lateral incisors and lower permanent central incisors.

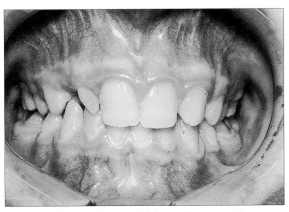

Fig. 8.2 Absence of upper left lateral incisor with suppression of the corresponding tooth on the other side.

permanent tooth may be approached in one of two ways. The deciduous tooth may be extracted and the space allowed to close, aided where necessary by appliance therapy. In this case, the earlier the deciduous tooth is extracted the better. Alternatively, the deciduous tooth may be retained as long as possible and the gap filled by a fixed or removable prosthesis or implant when it is eventually lost. If an implant is being considered, retention of the deciduous tooth until a late stage is important in maintaining the alveolar process.

Treatment decisions depend upon which tooth is missing, the amount of tooth substance available to close the space, the condition of the deciduous tooth and the occlusal relationship of the arches. In uncomplicated Class I occlusions, it is usually best to aim for space closure in order to avoid expensive artificial replacements which need maintenance for a lifetime. When the upper lateral incisors are missing, the canines usually develop in forward positions, simplifying space closure in the labial segment. The canine may be made to look more like a lateral incisor by reducing the height of the cusp but the cosmetic outcome may be limited by the dark yellow colour of the canine crown. Acid-etch additions to create an incisal edge are possible but veneering is limited by the bulbous nature of the canine crown. Mesial migration of upper buccal segments may be encouraged by extracting the upper second deciduous molars where the lateral incisors are missing. The intention of this artifice is to promote mesial drift of the permanent molars and mesial eruption of the premolars. A detailed consideration of treatment options when upper lateral incisors are absent is given by Millar and Taylor.[5] If lower second premolars are absent in a Class I occlusion, the second deciduous molars should be extracted at an early stage, but it will be necessary to compensate for this by extracting upper premolars at a later date (Fig. 8.3). It is also worth remembering that much anchorage is needed in closing the space occupied by a second deciduous molar because it is a large tooth and that late extraction of deciduous molars is followed by much tipping of the adjacent teeth.[6] Early extraction of the deciduous molar is desirable because it promotes space closure but on the other hand, it is possible that the related premolar is simply delayed in its development. Thus the clinician is faced with an enigmatic choice. On the one hand, he wants to extract the deciduous molar as early as possible if the premolar is absent, yet he must be sure that the premolar is absent before extracting the deciduous tooth. This author's personal cut off point is 8.5 years of age. If the premolar is not visible radiographically by this age, there is a reasonable certainty that it is not going to develop. Others use development of two thirds of the first premolar root as their critical stage.[7]

There may be a good case for artificial replacement of missing lower second premolars in a Class II malocclusion where the lower arch should be kept as big and as full as possible. Similarly, artificial replacement of missing lateral incisors may be appropriate in the upper arch of a Class III malocclusion where proclination of the upper labial segment is part of the treatment plan (Fig. 8.4). Spaces caused by missing upper laterals in Class II cases and missing lower second premolars in Class III cases may be used to treat the malocclusion.

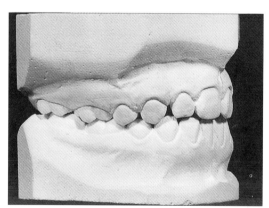

Fig. 8.3 Absence of lower second premolars compensated in the upper arch by extraction of second premolars without mechanical treatment.

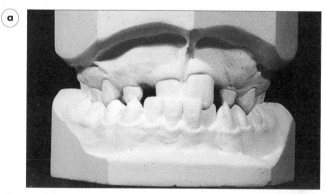

(a)

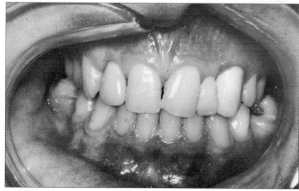

(b)

Fig. 8.4 Class III malocclusion with absence of upper left lateral incisor and conical lateral on the other side. Treatment consisted of alignment of incisors followed by crowning of the right lateral and artificial replacement of the left lateral. (a) before treatment (b) after treatment.

Some pioneering work in Scandinavia[8] has explored the possibilities of transplanting lower premolars into the place of missing upper incisors. Ideally, the root of the premolar should be one third to half formed at the time of transplantation. A success rate of over 90% is reported. The premolar is usually implanted with the buccal and lingual surfaces placed mesially and distally to facilitate subsequent crowning or placement of a veneer.

Extra teeth

Extra teeth are found in the permanent dentitions of between 1.6 and 2.1% of British children depending on the age group investigated. Males are affected more frequently than females.[9] Extra teeth may be classified as: supplemental, which resemble a tooth of the normal series in size and form; supernumerary, which are clearly recognisable as teeth but would not be mistaken for a tooth of the normal series; and odontomes, where there are multiple small teeth or an irregular mass of dental tissue. All three varieties may be found in the incisor, canine, premolar and molar areas of both jaws with the exception that supplemental upper canines do not seem to exist.

A supplemental lateral incisor may appear in the line of the arch or on the lingual or palatal side of the arch (Fig. 8.5). It is frequently difficult to decide which is the lateral incisor and which is the supplemental tooth, which leaves a free choice of the tooth to be extracted as treatment of the almost inevitable crowding. Rarely, both the lateral incisor and the supplemental tooth may be retained or the extra tooth extracted and transplanted to another position in the mouth (Fig. 8.6) A supernumerary tooth is often found near the upper mid-line where it is called a mesiodens. A mesiodens may erupt in the line of the arch (Fig. 8.7) or may be sufficiently far from the teeth of the normal series that it can be ignored (Fig. 8.8) More commonly, mesiodentes are palatally placed in relation to the upper central incisors and may be associated with delayed eruption or rotation of a central incisor or a midline diastema. Those associated with delayed eruption are often large, tuberculate, and have incomplete root formation. Conical mesiodentes are more frequently associated with rotation or a diastema.[10] Rarely, a conical supernumerary tooth may be fused to the central incisor (Fig. 8.9).

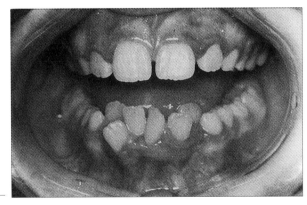

Fig. 8.5 Supplemental lower incisors.

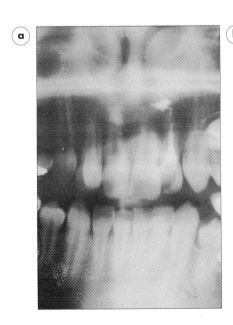

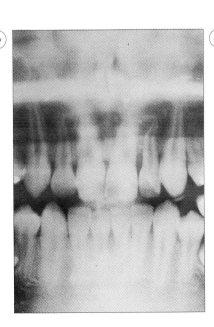

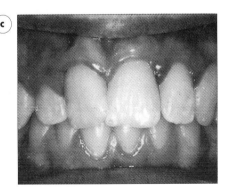

Fig. 8.6 (a) Radiograph showing supplemental upper right lateral incisor superimposed on the corresponding tooth of the normal series. The prognosis for the upper left lateral incisor is poor. (b) supplemental tooth extracted and transplanted into the socket of the upper left lateral incisor (c) clinical view after transplantation.

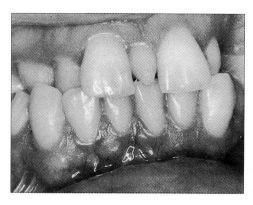

Fig. 8.7 Mesiodens erupted in the line of the arch.

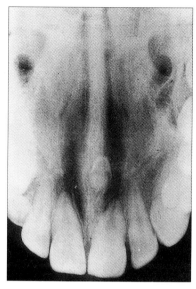

Fig. 8.8 Mesiodens far away from teeth of the normal series.

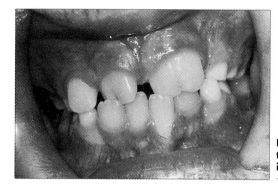

Fig. 8.9 Conical supernumerary tooth fused with an upper central incisor.

A fixed appliance is usually needed for the correction of rotations and any midline diastema after extraction of the supernumerary tooth. Opinions vary on the best approach to delayed eruption. Some authorities remove the supernumerary tooth and expose the central incisor, packing the wound open. The labial flap may be repositioned apically so as to give a gingival margin of attached mucosa. This is almost invariably followed by unaided eruption of the incisor over the next 2 years (Fig. 8.10).[11] Other surgeons remove the supernumerary tooth together with some bone and close the wound. This is done on the grounds that a more healthy gingival margin will result.[12] A bracket attached to a piece of gold chain may be bonded to the central incisor at the time of operation. Bringing the chain through the wound allows traction to be applied to the unerupted tooth. Effective bonding of a bracket in the usual position at the time of operation is not easy and requires extensive removal of bone to permit access to the labial surface of the tooth. Some authorities use custom-made attachments[13] and an incisal bracket has been described to meet this problem.[14] Closure of the wound without traction is followed by eruption of the central incisor in about 78% of cases.[15] A second surgical procedure, which may be quite minor, is needed for exposure in the unerupted remainder. All authorities agree that early interceptive treatment has great benefits in delayed eruption. In patients who are not treated until a late stage, there is a tendency for root formation

of the unerupted incisor to continue in the absence of eruption so that the root apex on the affected side is at a higher level and it may be dilacerated.[16]

Removal of large odontomes in the incisor region leave large deficiencies in the bone, but alignment of the incisors is usually possible (Fig. 8.11).

Supernumerary teeth in the upper canine region are common in cleft palate but rare in non-cleft subjects. When they occur, the eruption of the canine is usually delayed (Fig. 8.12). Sizeable odontomes occur in the lower canine region and occasionally one finds a collection of denticles on the lingual side of a lower canine. The latter rarely affects teeth of the normal series (Fig. 8.13).

In some parts of the world supplemental teeth are quite common in the premolar region, where they usually erupt on the lingual side of the arch (Fig. 8.14). Conical supernumeraries and odontomes in the premolar region are less frequent and may develop some time after full eruption of the premolar teeth (Fig. 8.15).[17]

Supplemental molars are not uncommon. On the whole, supernumeraries in the molar and premolar areas have little effect upon the teeth of the normal series except that delayed eruption of a second molar may be one of the first signs of a denticle occlusal to it (Fig. 8.16). Odontomes are less frequent and may delay eruption of a molar. Eruption of the molar is possible following removal of the odontome (Fig. 8.17).

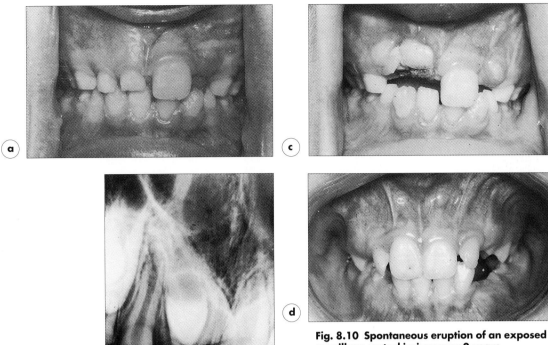

Fig. 8.10 Spontaneous eruption of an exposed maxillary central incisor over 2 years.
(a) delayed eruption of the upper right central incisor with retention of the corresponding deciduous tooth.
(b) radiograph showing supernumerary tooth in close relation to the delayed central incisor. (c) following removal of the supernumerary tooth and exposure of the central incisor. (d) 2 years later – note the gingival levels.

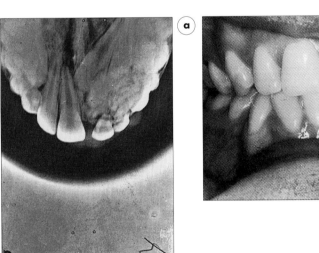

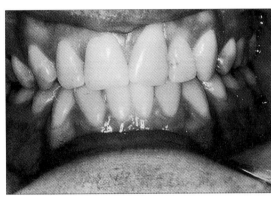

Fig. 8.11 (a) Odontome in the upper incisor region with delayed eruption of a central and lateral incisor.
(b) following removal of the odontome and alignment of the incisors with a fixed appliance.

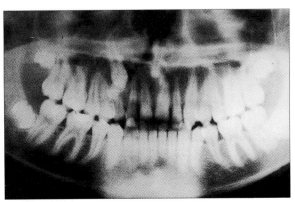

Fig. 8.12 Conical supernumerary tooth in the upper right canine region associated with delayed eruption of the canine.

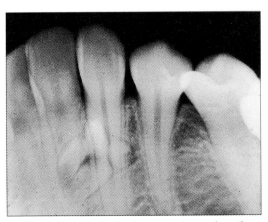

Fig. 8.13 Denticles in the lower canine region. These are invariably on the lingual side of the arch.

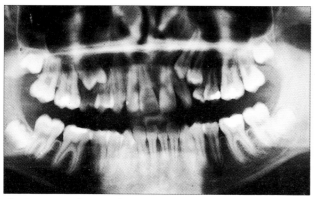

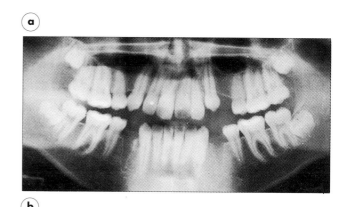

Fig. 8.14 Supplemental upper premolars. There is a supplemental premolar in both upper quadrants.

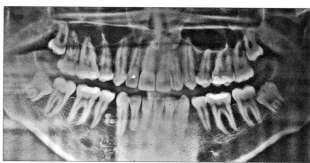

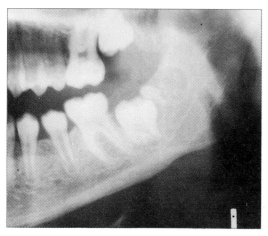

Fig. 8.16 Conical supernumerary tooth associated with delayed eruption of lower second molar.

Fig. 8.15 Late-developing supernumerary teeth in the lower right premolar region. (a) age 13 years (b) age 15 years.

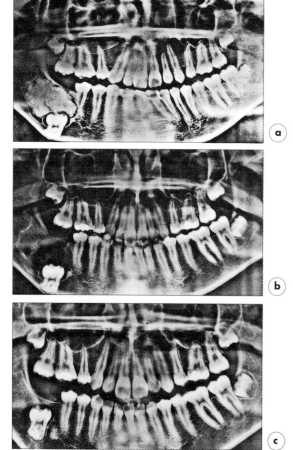

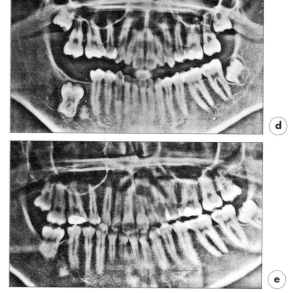

Fig. 8.17 Eruption of a submerged lower molar following removal of an odontome. (a) age 13 years: There is a large odontome in the lower right molar region and delayed eruption of the only molar tooth in that quadrant (b) immediately after removal of the odontome (c) age 14 years: some intra-osseous eruption of the molar has occurred (d) age 15 years: eruption has continued (e) age 16 years: the molar tooth has erupted to the general occlusal level.

Interceptive treatment gives the best hope of success in most of these cases. Dentistry must rely on general practitioners and dentists in the Community Service for early detection. This depends on nothing more complicated than counting the teeth and comparing the findings with the typical child of the same age.

A system of patient examination in relation to interception is described in Chapter 9.

Early loss of deciduous teeth

Premature loss of deciduous teeth, particularly deciduous molars, may have effects on the underlying premolar, on the other teeth in the same arch and on teeth in the opposing arch.

The traditional teaching is that very early extraction of a deciduous molar may lead to delayed eruption of the permanent successor because dense cortical bone and fibrous tissue is formed in the extraction site. While recent work has cast doubt on this aspect,[18] all authorities seem to agree that extraction of a deciduous molar shortly before the premolar is ready to erupt hastens eruption of the permanent tooth.[19]

The effect of premature loss of deciduous teeth on the contiguous teeth in the same arch has been largely covered in the discussion of crowding. Where there is an innate tendency towards crowding, loss of a deciduous molar leads to space closure partly by mesial movement of teeth behind the extraction site and partly by distal movement of more anterior teeth. The latter may lead to movement of the midline towards the site of the extraction.

Enforced extraction of a deciduous molar where space maintenance is not practicable or desirable raises the question of a balancing extraction from the other side of the same arch to maintain the midline and a compensating extraction from the opposing arch to maintain the occlusion, bearing in mind that subsequent extraction of premolars will be an almost inevitable consequence. Maintenance of the midline and occlusion is a desirable and attainable objective in Class I malocclusion but not in Class II or Class III cases where appliance therapy will be required in any event. In Class II cases, keeping the lower arch as large as possible and not allowing overmuch space closure in the upper arch are at least as important as maintaining the midline so that neither balancing nor compensating extractions are desirable, no matter which deciduous molar must be extracted. In Class III cases a generous upper arch is important so that balancing extractions are not desirable in the upper arch and balancing or compensating extractions in the lower arch would have little effect because the mandible is usually so large that little space closure occurs.

Extraction of an upper first deciduous molar in a Class I malocclusion should be balanced by extracting the first deciduous molar on the other side but not compensated for in the lower arch. Extraction of a lower first deciduous molar in a Class I malocclusion calls for a balancing extraction on the other side and compensating extractions in the upper arch. Unless the extraction is very early, loss of a second deciduous molar has little effect on the midline so that balancing and compensating extractions are rarely necessary.

In summary, the only indications for balancing or compensating extractions are in Class I cases, i.e. balancing first deciduous molar extractions in either arch and compensating for lower first deciduous molar extractions by extracting the opposing tooth. If an upper D must be removed, two teeth come out, if a lower D must be removed, four teeth come out.

Over-eruption of opposing deciduous molars is rarely a problem because the deciduous molars will have run out of eruption potential before the extraction in most cases.

Whether the lower permanent incisors, deprived by extraction of support from the buccal segments, develop in a more lingual position than would otherwise be the case has not been proven but extrapolation from the work of Mills[20] suggests that this effect has been exaggerated in the classical teaching of the past.

Prolonged retention of deciduous teeth

Bearing in mind that all unerupted teeth are surrounded by a resorptive follicle, it seems unlikely that the roots of retained deciduous teeth could cause much deflection of the permanent successors at an early stage of development.

A much more likely explanation of a 'double row of teeth' is that the permanent teeth were out of line from the start and have failed to resorb the baby teeth. After eruption of the permanent teeth, however, contact between the crowns of deciduous and permanent teeth may prevent spontaneous alignment of the permanent series. The retained deciduous teeth should be extracted and at least some improvement in permanent tooth alignment can be confidently predicted (Fig. 8.18). A special case of retained deciduous teeth is the so-called submerged deciduous molar which is sometimes associated with absence of the corresponding premolar (Fig. 8.19). These deciduous teeth are not really submerged in the sense that they have sunk down into the bone. The true explanation is that they have remained in a fairly constant vertical position while the adjacent teeth and alveolar processes have grown up round them. Ankylosis, which often occurs round those submerged teeth, is best detected by percussing the tooth with the mirror handle when the note will be heard reverberating through the bone. Sometimes these teeth may become completely

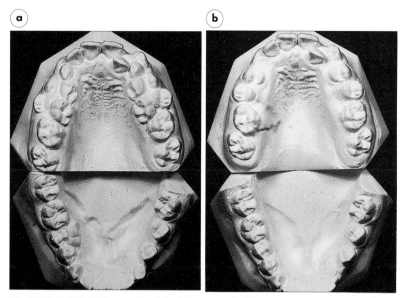

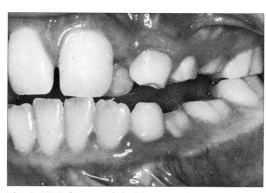

Fig. 8.19 Submerged deciduous molars.

Fig. 8.18 (a) Multiple retained deciduous teeth. (b) spontaneous improvement of permanent teeth following removal of retained teeth.

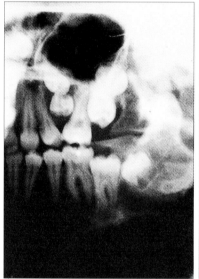

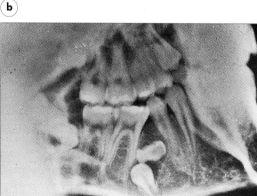

Fig. 8.20 Completely submerged deciduous molars with delayed eruption of the corresponding premolar. (a) in the upper arch (b) in the lower arch.

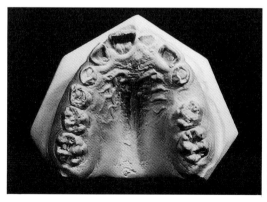

Fig. 8.21 Incisive papilla at an angle to mid-palatal raphe following loss of an upper central incisor and drifting of the other central incisor towards the side where the tooth has been lost.

submerged and more or less resorbed (Fig. 8.20). Parents and students may be impressed by the diagnosis of a completely submerged second deciduous molar on clinical examination alone. The clue is a first permanent molar which is very mesially inclined, like a small child tripping over a football, with the apex well spaced from the first premolar.

The traditional treatment of partially sub-merged deciduous molars is extraction[21] but this must be followed by prolonged wearing of space maintainers with the risk of decalcification and soft tissue problems. There is more recent evidence that patience is rewarded by natural exfoliation in most cases.[22,23] Of course, the dentist must guard against the teeth becoming completely submerged. A vigilant wait and watch policy is appropriate.

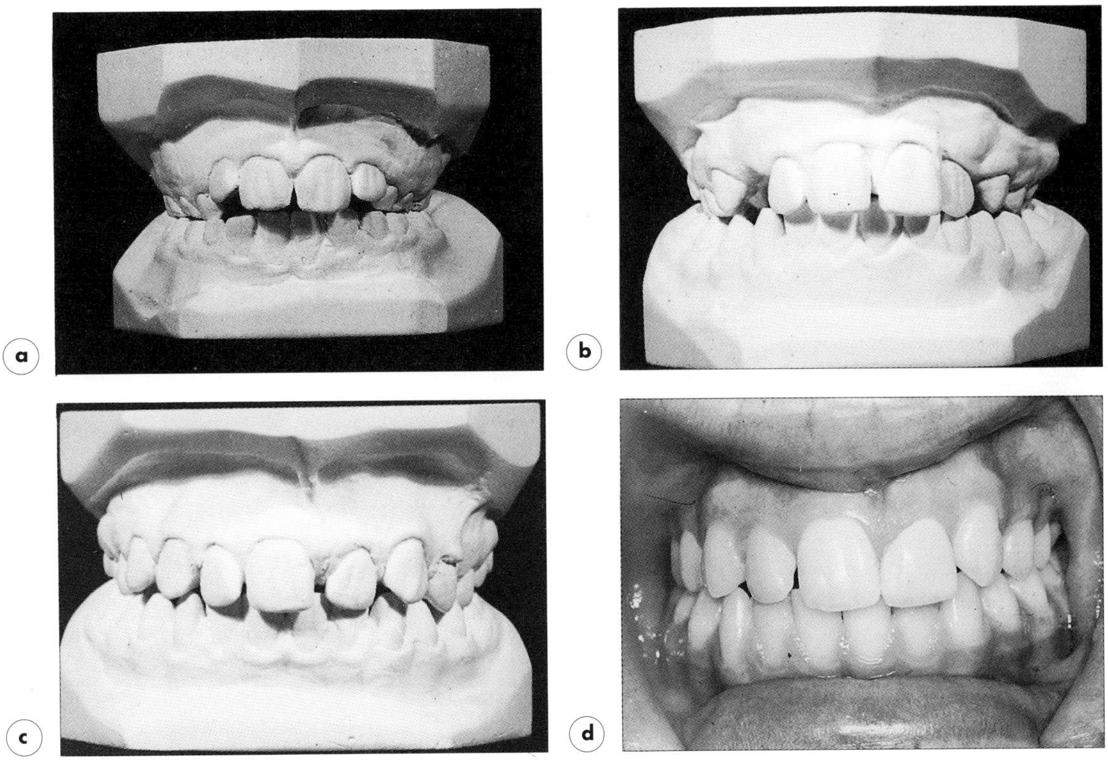

Fig. 8.22 (a) Class II division 1 malocclusion prior to orthodontic treatment. (b) Upper left central incisor lost traumatically. Prosthetic replacement by general practitioner. (c) partial upper denture withdrawn and orthodontic treatment (d) crown restoration of lateral incisor to simulate central incisor.

Loss of permanent teeth

Trauma during contact sports or precipitate descent from bicycles is the most frequent cause of central incisor tooth loss in children. Children with increased overjet and incompetent lips seem particularly vulnerable.[24–26] Unilateral loss of an incisor is almost invariably followed by a shift of the mid-line into the space. If incisor teeth drift they take the incisive papilla with them so that midline shift can be identified by an angle between the incisive papilla and the mid-palatal raphe (Fig. 8.21).

In these circumstances, it is frequently difficult to decide whether the spaces should be maintained by a removable prosthesis with a view to bridgework or implant, or whether it is best to allow some space closure, make the lateral incisor more upright and then modify its shape with a crown or veneer to match the central on the other side. Bridgework may give the best aesthetic result at the expense of sound tooth substance involved in the abutments. Placing a crown or a veneer on the lateral incisor involves less preparation, but it may be difficult to produce a good mesial contact area while at the same time avoiding a ledge at the mesial gingival margin. A fixed appliance can ease this problem by setting the lateral incisor upright in the middle of the space.

Each case must be treated on its merits, the crucial points being whether the shift in the midline is acceptable and whether it is necessary to extract premolars to make space for a full-sized replacement for the lost incisor. There is at least one orthodontist who favours crowning the lateral incisor as it is likely to result in a more enduring and trouble-free

dentition (Fig. 8.22). It must be admitted, however, that the advent of bonded bridges favours the bridgework side of the argument. Rarely, a premolar tooth may be transplanted into the position of a lost central incisor[8].

Impaction

Dental impaction means that a tooth has driven into, or is pressed firmly against, another tooth. Impaction is often applied to unerupted maxillary canines but in many cases the canine is not impacted against another tooth and such terms as bony impaction are difficult to sustain. Accordingly, delayed eruption of the maxillary canine will be considered under the heading of delayed eruption.

Canines excepted, the teeth most commonly impacted are third molars, second premolars and occasionally, upper first molars.

Impaction of third molars

Impaction of third molars is a sequel of crowding. This crowding may be treated interceptively by extraction of the third molar itself or by other teeth in the same quadrant as described in Chapter 7. As far as the third molar itself is concerned, opinion has swung away from prophylactic removal because it is now thought that many third molars removed in the past (at vast expense to the Health Service or the patients) would have remained free of related symptoms. Balancing cost, anaesthetic and surgical risks and morbidity following surgery against the probability of symptoms in the future, opinion seems to favour third molar removal only where there are clear indications such as pericoronitis, relevant caries or root resorption of the second molars, cysts, tumours or destruction of adjacent teeth and bone.[27] Of course, the decision may be dominated by non-dental factors such as the patient going on a polar expedition, emigrating to a remote area or serving in the armed forces during a war when prophylactic removal may be appropriate.

The question of whether lower third molars contribute to crowding of other teeth in the lower arch of the average patient is not simple, and in the individual patient it is very complex. All other things being equal, in the average patient, the presence of third molars seems to be associated with greater crowding of other teeth in the lower arch.[28] The problem for the individual patient is that all other things are never equal and that he is unlikely to conform to the average. Other variables, such as extraction of other teeth, degree of overbite, facial growth, growth rotations, muscular forces and the anterior component of force, soft tissue changes and periodontal support all seem to play a part in late lower arch crowding or its absence. In some ways, the debate is reminiscent of arguments in the ENT literature relating to the once-fashionable removal of tonsils, or to extraction of first molars discussed in Chapter 7. At one time, prophylactic removal of third molars was in vogue but it is now realised that extraction of third molars is not a panacea against late lower arch crowding which can be treated more positively by other means if it does occur. The other side of the question, which is rarely discussed, is whether treatment of lower arch crowding is an effective prophylaxis against third molar impaction. Here orthodontics is on more sure ground. There is ample evidence that decisive treatment of crowding by extraction of almost any tooth (without appliance therapy) has a favourable influence on the eruption of third molars and that the degree of success improves the further distally the extraction is carried out.[29] Extraction of second molars will almost invariably allow eruption of third molars, most of them in good or acceptable positions.[30]

Impaction of second premolars

Impaction of second premolars is almost invariably a sequel of premature loss of second deciduous molars which may be treated interceptively by space maintenance or timely extractions.

Impaction of first molars

A rather rare but interesting impaction is the upper first permanent molar which becomes lodged above the distal bulge of the second deciduous molar (Fig. 8.23). According to Bennett[1] this is a local abnormality, but some orthodontists see it as a sign of crowding in the molar region. Impactions of this kind often resolve spontaneously (the so-called 'jump' cases) whereas others need some treatment (the 'hold' cases). The chances of a first molar disimpacting spontaneously diminish greatly after 7–8 years of age.[31] The approach to 'hold' cases depends upon whether the orthodontist is a follower of Bennett or not. If so, he will thread a piece of 0.6mm soft brass wire from buccal to lingual above the mesial contact area of the first molar and twist the ends together tightly on the occlusal side of the contact area. This may generate sufficient pressure to move the molar the small distance required to effect disimpaction, but it may be a difficult procedure. Alternatively, a spring on a removable appliance may be engaged on a blob of composite resin or small metal attachment bonded to the tooth. Some clinicians use headgear to ease the molar distally.

If, on the other hand, the orthodontist believes that the impaction is a sign of crowding, he will extract the second deciduous molar, allow eruption of the permanent molar and treat the crowding later by extraction of a premolar tooth.

Delayed eruption

Abnormally delayed eruption of many teeth suggests a generalised retardation of growth as in the endocrinopathies or a syndromal condition such as osteopetrosis, Down's syndrome or cleidocranial dysplasia. More localised causes such as impaction, supernumerary teeth and dilaceration are described under the appropriate heading.

Delayed eruption of the maxillary canine is a frequent problem in orthodontic practice. It seems to occur in about 3% of the adult population.[32] The upper canine starts to calcify during the first year of life and has a long descent to the level of occlusion. For normal eruption it must move from a lingual developmental position to the buccal side of the arch through cramped surroundings and the fact that it erupts after

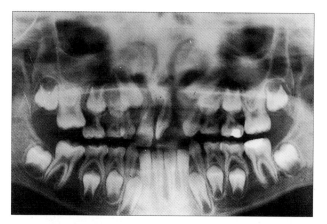

Fig. 8.23 Upper right first permanent molar impacted against second deciduous molar. The resorption of the second deciduous molar on the left side may be a sign that the first permanent molar was similarly impacted and spontaneous correction has occurred. The patient has a unilateral cleft palate.

the lateral incisor and first premolar means that it is liable to suffer from crowding. Canines which erupt normally usually move in a palatal direction up to age 9 years and then move buccally up to the time of eruption.[33] On average, there is a difference of 5mm between the most palatal position of a canine and its most buccal position 1 year after eruption. Most eruptive movement occurs between ages 9–12 years. Most canines which are delayed in their eruption fail to make the crossing from the palatal to labial side of the arch and remain palatally placed. From this position the pointed tooth continues to move palatally and seems to track along the line of palatal periosteum behind the lateral and central incisors so that the already abnormal situation becomes even worse.[34] Resorption of the lateral and even the central incisor may occur. Although crowding and local conditions may contribute to the aetiology of delayed canines, it has been pointed out that palatal positioning and delayed eruption of canines may occur in arches which are spaced, that the condition runs in families and that there is frequently an abnormality of the lateral incisor which may take the form of invagination, reduced size or absence.[35,36] This collection of factors argues in favour of a developmental syndrome of which an ectopic position of the developing canine may be a manifestation. Some authors have gone so far as to suggest that delayed eruption of maxillary canines may be a microform of clefting.[37] Zilberman et al[36] point out that delayed root development of a diminutive lateral incisor may be a mechanical factor in failing to guide the canine into position.

Ericson and Kürol[38] have shown that extraction of the deciduous canine between ages 10 and 13 years can be a very effective treatment for palatally placed permanent canines. The success rate for this procedure is 91% if the unerupted canine overlaps the lateral incisor by less than half of the breadth of the root on a pantomograph. The success rate is 64% if the overlap is greater (Fig. 8.24). Power and Short[39] have shown that these favourable results occur only where there is sufficient space in the arch to accommodate the permanent canine.

If the maxillary canines are not palpable in the buccal sulcus after the age of 10 years their positions should be investigated radiographically as described in Chapter 3 and the deciduous canines removed if the permanent teeth are found to be palatally placed.

Overall, the treatment options for ectopic canines are the interceptive extraction of deciduous canines, extraction of the permanent canine, exposure of the canine with orthodontic alignment (making space as required), surgical repositioning of the unerupted canine, allowing the canine to erupt in place of a resorbed or otherwise pathological lateral incisor, or accepting the situation with regular review.

There are 396 combinations of variables in making treatment decisions, all of which are covered in the computer programme available from the author*.

Teeth of abnormal form

In the present context there is no need to cover the full breadth and depth of the bizarre but only those abnormalities which offer some precognition of a developing malocclusion

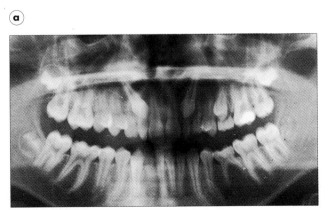
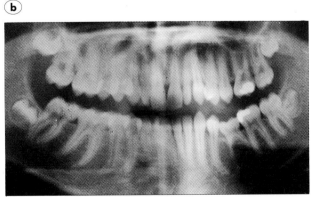

Fig. 8.24 Spontaneous eruption of maxillary canines following extraction of deciduous canines. (a) before extractions: the permanent canines overlap the lateral incisors by the full breadth of the lateral incisor roots. (b) after extractions: the canines have erupted into good alignment. The lower left second premolar is absent.

and those where early treatment may be an advantage.

Gemination between two deciduous incisors is usually followed by absence of a permanent tooth. Gemination between a lower deciduous canine and lateral incisor is invariably followed by absence of the lower lateral incisor. Early detection and early removal of such geminated teeth is usually rewarded by eruption of the permanent canines in forward positions and space closure (Fig. 8.25). Gemination between a deciduous incisor and a supernumerary element may presage a supernumerary permanent tooth, a permanent tooth of abnormal form or there may be no abnormality. Gemination or connation of permanent incisors may be treated by aligning the abnormally formed teeth. In most cases, reduction of the number of teeth in the arch will be necessary. The abnormal tooth may be masked by acid-etch restoration or by milling a groove in the labial enamel to make it look like two teeth. In some cases the abnormal crown may be split and part of it removed.[40] In gross abnormalities, extraction is the only option (Fig. 8. 26).

Apart from enamel hypoplasia, which can usually be treated conservatively, the abnormality of crown form most frequently encountered by the orthodontist is the conical or feline upper lateral incisor. This may be associated with absence of the corresponding tooth on the other side. Conical lateral incisors frequently have an invagination or dens in dente and may be associated with misplaced maxillary canine teeth. Such conical teeth may be treated by extraction and space closure, extraction and prosthetic replacement or by retaining the abnormal tooth and building it up to a more normal size. In many cases, this is difficult because the neck of the tooth is so small.

Dilaceration of a permanent incisor may follow trauma to the corresponding deciduous tooth or it may be of unknown aetiology. Orthodontic alignment of these teeth is usually possible.

Abnormal labial fraenum

The presence of a large and fleshy fraenum is often associated with a diastema between the upper central incisors. On the other hand, it is

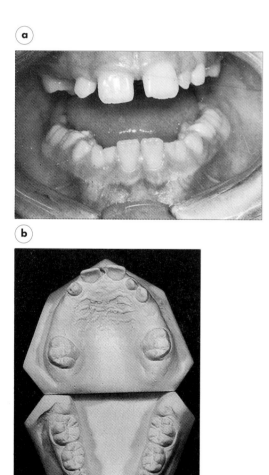

Fig. 8.25 (a) Geminated lower deciduous canine and lateral incisor. (b) eruption of permanent canines in forward positions following removal of geminated teeth.

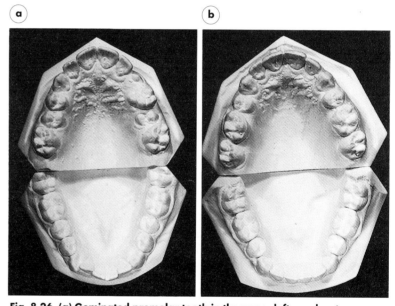

Fig. 8.26 (a) Geminated premolar tooth in the upper left quadrant. (b) alignment with fixed appliance following extraction. A premolar was extracted from each of the other quadrants.

possible to find large fraena with no mid-line diastema and mid-line diastemata with only a small fraenum (Fig. 8.27). The current concept is that, in a spaced arch, a large fraenum will cause the space to appear in the mid-line.[41] If the fraenum is not so prominent, the spacing will be more evenly distributed between the teeth. A prominent intermaxillary suture may also be a minor factor.[42]

Even though a direct cause-and-effect relationship between fraena and diastemata is not proven, a prominent fraenum interrupts the transseptal fibres between the central incisors[43] and it is best to excise the fraenum if a large diastema is to be closed. Contraction of scar tissue following fraenectomy tends to draw the central incisors together, thus facilitating or even eliminating the need for appliance therapy. Opinions vary on whether the fraenectomy should be performed before or after closure of the diastema. Surgeons usually prefer to do the fraenectomy early for reasons of access.

Upper mid-line diastema
A space or diastema between the upper central incisors when they first erupt is not unusual and may be associated with other features of the 'ugly duckling' stage. The majority of these spaces close spontaneously through time. In some, closure does not occur until 19 years of age.[44] Clues to the spaces which will close spontaneously are the age of the child, the size of the space and the mesio-distal inclinations of the central incisors. Distally inclined incisors are more likely to move mesially. Before giving assurances of spontaneous correction, however, it is important to confirm that the upper lateral incisors are present and that there is no pathological entity, such as a cyst or supernumerary tooth, occupying space between the central incisor roots.

Other causes of mid-line diastema are proclination of upper incisors or a familial or racial tendency towards a spaced dentition. In some parts of Africa a midline diastema is regarded as beautiful and a useful way of feeding in case of tetanus.[45] Most Caucasian patients, however, are unimpressed by this argument and find a mid-line diastema cosmetically disadvantageous.

While a small diastema can be closed with a removable appliance, larger spaces are best managed with fixed appliances which offer the facility of approximating the roots as well as the crowns. If a mid-line diastema is to be closed and kept closed, the central incisors need to be supported in mesial positions. Bonded retainers can be helpful but the most satisfactory way of enhancing stability is to close all spaces in the upper arch by mesial movement of teeth round the arch or by retroclining the incisors if the overjet is increased. In some cases, reduction of the lower arch perimeter will assist retroclination in the upper. In many instances it is necessary to provide artificial tooth substance to produce firm approximal contacts. This can be done by crowning, veneering or making additions to the central or lateral incisors. A fixed or removable prosthesis is required if the spaces are excessively large or if the lateral incisors are absent.

Habits
The sucking of fingers or a thumb often produces a malocclusion. On the other hand, there are many children who suck a digit without any apparent effect on the dentition. The determining factors are the frequency, intensity and duration of the habit and the way in which the digit is inserted. The finding that all dummy-sucking ceased by age 2.5 years whereas about half of digit-suckers continued up to age 8 years has led to the suggestion that children should be encouraged to suck a dummy.[46]

In its classic form, the malocclusion produced by digit-sucking is proclination and spacing of upper incisors[47] and an anterior open bite which can be distinguished from open bites of other aetiology by the fact that it is almost invariably asymmetrical. There may be contraction of the upper arch and a unilateral crossbite.[48] If this kind of malocclusion exists, the dentist may be absolutely certain that the child is indulging in a habit.

The reasons for digit-sucking are summarised

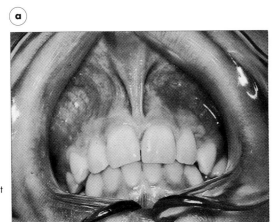
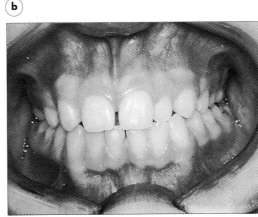

Fig. 8.27 (a) large fraenum but no diastema. (b) diastema but small fraenum. The upper right lateral incisor is absent creating a spacing tendency.

in a recent briefing paper[49] and are beyond the scope of this book except to the extent that they relate to treatment.

No one likes being told what to do. Children must get fed up with being badgered about their behaviour and if they happen to suck a thumb it is a cast-iron certainty that they will have been repeatedly reminded of it before they reach the dentist. Children should be told in a matter-of-fact way that they are sucking a thumb, rather than being asked whether they do so.

The approach to treatment should be equally matter-of-fact: 'You are not going to suck your thumb for the rest of your life so why don't you stop today.' The long-term success rate for this approach is very high. If, after 6 months, the child is having difficulty in stopping a habit, a simple appliance with an inverted goalpost may be provided to help him on his way (Fig. 8.28). Following cessation of the habit, the associated malocclusion will usually resolve spontaneously (Fig. 8.29), but it is worth remembering that there may be other features of the occlusion which are not related to the habit and may benefit from orthodontic treatment. Likewise, thrusting of the tongue into the open bite is likely to disappear on cessation of the habit but may perpetuate the open bite in the rare circumstance that it is endogenous. Tongue function may improve after orthodontic correction of the incisor relationship.[50]

Ectopic position of the tooth germ

An ectopic position really means that none of the well-recognised aetiological factors seem to be operating and it is assumed that the tooth was out of line from the start or 'just grew that way'. It would be difficult to believe that the presence of a canine low in the symphysis, as shown in Figure 8.30, could have arisen in any other way. A degree of ectopia must also contribute to many of the other abnormalities in this chapter such as transposition, impacted upper first molars and delayed eruption of the maxillary canine.

Transposition

True transposition, i.e. complete bodily switching of two teeth, must be extremely rare but some degree of transposition involving the crowns of the teeth is more common. Transposition occurs most frequently between the upper canine and first premolar but it is also seen between the upper canine and lateral incisor and between the lower lateral incisor and canine (Fig. 8.31). Lower canines have even been known to cross the midline and erupt between the lateral incisor and canine on the other side.[51]

Those occurring in the upper arch are usually best treated by completing the transposition with fixed appliances. Minor degrees of transposition involving the lower lateral incisor and canine can be corrected if seen early. Later correction often leaves a dehiscence on the lingual side of the lateral incisor. In the interceptive field, extraction of the lateral incisor may provide a simple and effective solution when the child is seen early enough and there is sufficient crowding to assist closure of the extraction space.

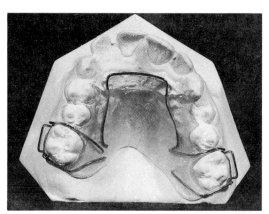

Fig. 8.28 'Goalpost' appliance to help the patient abandon a thumb-sucking habit.

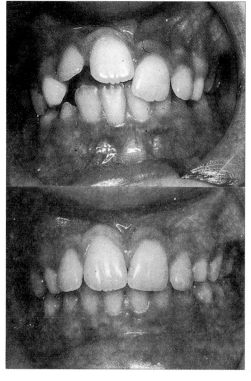

Fig. 8.29 Spontaneous correction of anterior open bite following cessation of a thumbsucking habit.

Pathology

Early recognition and early referral is the best service that the practitioner can give in cases where pathological lesions, such as cysts, tumours and odontomes interfere with the eruption of teeth or cause displacement of teeth of the normal series.

As in all aspects of interceptive orthodontics, a sound knowledge of normal occlusal development is the key to early recognition and to early and effective treatment or referral to the appropriate specialist.

*Guidelines on treatment of unerupted maxillary canines computed by Andrew Richardson and Terry Gregg.

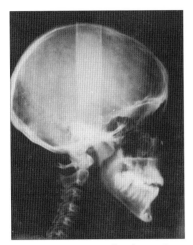

Fig. 8.30 An example of ectopic position of the tooth germ. A lower canine is placed at the lower border of the mandibular symphysis.

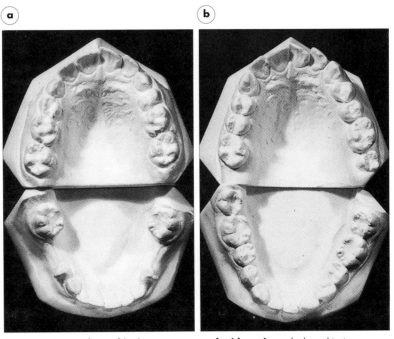

Fig. 8.31 Lower lateral incisors transposed with canines: the lateral incisors were extracted, (a) age 10 years, (b) age 20 years.

References

1 Bennett Sir N. *The science and practice of dental surgery.* p. 201. London: Waverley, 1931.

2 Bjerklin K, Kürol J, Valentin J. Ectopic eruption of maxillary first permanent molars and association with other tooth and developmental disturbances. *Eur J Orthod* 1992; **14**: 369–375.

3 Davies PL. Agenesis of teeth of the permanent dentition. A frequency study in Sydney schoolchildren. *Aust Dent J* 1968; **13**: 146–150.

4 Dermaut LR, Goeffers KR, De Smit AA. Prevalence of tooth agenesis correlated with jaw relationship and dental crowding. *Am J Orthod Dentofac Orthop* 1986; **90**: 204–210.

5 Millar BJ, Taylor NG. Lateral thinking: the management of missing upper lateral incisors. *Br Dent J* 1995; **179**: 99–106.

6 Lindqvist B. Extraction of the deciduous second molar in hypodontia. *Eur J Orthod* 1980; **2**: 173–181.

7 Joondeph DR, McNeill RW. Congenitally absent second premolars: an interceptive approach. *Am J Orthod* 1971; **59**: 50–66.

8 Andreasen JO, Paulsen HU, Yu Z, Ahlquist R, Bayer T, Schwartz O. A long-term study of 370 autotransplanted premolars. *Eur J Orthod* 1990; **12**: Part 1: 3–13, Part 11: 14–24, Part III: 25–37, Part IV: 38–50.

9 Brook AH. Dental anomalies of number, form and size: their prevalence in British schoolchildren. *J Int Assoc Dent Children* 1974; **5**: 37–53.

10 De Biase DD. Midline supernumeraries and eruption of the maxillary central incisor. *Dent Practit* 1969; **20**: 35–40.

11 Burke P. The eruptive movements of permanent central incisor teeth after surgical exposure. *Eur Orthod Soc Trans* 1963: 251–262.

12 Wong-Lee TK, Wong FCK. Maintaining an ideal tooth-gingiva relationship when exposing and aligning an impacted tooth. *Br J Orthod* 1985; **12**: 189–192.

13 Becker A. *The orthodontic treatment of impacted teeth.* London: Martin Dunitz Limited 1997.

14 Harrison M, Longhurst P. The incisal edge bracket for gold chain attachment to unerupted teeth. *Br J Orthod* 1998; **25**: 261–262.

15 Mitchell L, Bennett TG. Supernumerary teeth causing delayed eruption - a retrospective study. *Br J Orthod* 1992; **19**: 41–46.

16 Linehan CF, Richardson A. Delayed eruption of upper central incisor teeth. *J Irish Dent Assoc* 1967; **13**: 106–110.

17 Connolly IH. Richardson A. Late developing odontome in the lower premolar area - The enigmatic variations. *J Irish Dent Assoc* 1992; **38**: 21–23.

18 Bodegom IC. *Experiments on tooth eruption in miniature pigs.* Nijmegen: Drukkery Gebr Janssen N V, 1969.

19 Kerr WJS. The effects of the premature loss of deciduous canines and molars on the eruption of their successors. *Eur J Orthod* 1980; **2**: 123–128.

20 Mills JRE. The stability of the lower labial segment. *Dental Practit* 1968; **1**: 293–306.

21 Rygh P and Reitan K. Changes in the supporting tissues of submerged deciduous molars with and without permanent successors. *Eur Orthod Soc Trans* 1963; 171–184.

22 Kürol J, Koch G. The effect of extraction of infraoccluded deciduous molars: a longitudinal study. *Am J Orthod* 1985; **87**: 46–55.

23 Kürol J and Thilander B. Infraocclusion of primary molars and the effect on occlusal development, a longitudinal

study. *Eur J Orthod* 1984; **6**: 277–293.

24 Järvinen S. Incisal overjet and traumatic injuries to upper permanent incisors. A retrospective study. *Acta Odont Scand* 1978; **36**: 359–362.

25 Järvinen S. Traumatic injuries to upper permanent incisors related to age and incisal overjet. A retrospective study. *Acta Odont Scand* 1979; **37**: 335–338.

26 Burden DJ. An investigation of the association between overjet size, lip coverage. and traumatic injury to maxillary incisors. *Eur J Orthod* 1995; **17**: 513–517.

27 NIH Consensus development conference for removal of third molars. *J Oral Surg* 1980; **38**: 235–236.

28 Richardson ME. Late lower arch crowding: facial growth or forward drift? *Eur J Orthod* 1979; **1**: 219–25.

29 Richardson ME. The relative effect of the extraction of various teeth on the development of mandibular third molars. *Eur Orthod Soc Trans* 1975; 79–85.

30 Richardson ME, Richardson A. Lower third molar development subsequent to second molar extraction. *Am J Orthod Dentofac Orthop* 1993; **104**: 566–574.

31 Bjerklin K, Kürol J. Ectopic eruption of the maxillary first permanent molars: Etiologic factors. *Am J Orthod* 1983; **84**: 147–155.

32 Aitsalo K, Lehtincn R, Okcsala E. An orthopantomographic study of prevalence of impacted teeth. *Int J Oral Surg* 1972; **1**: 117–120.

33 Coulter J, Richardson A. Normal eruption of the maxillary canine quantified in three dimensions. *Eur J Orthod* 1997; **19**: 171–183.

34 McSherry P, Richardson A. Ectopic Eruption of the maxillary canine quantified in three dimensions. *Eur J Orthod* 1999; **21**: 41–48.

35 Richardson A, McKay C. Delayed eruption of maxillary canine teeth. Part 1 aetiology and diagnosis. *Proc Br Paedodont Soc* 1982; **12**: 15–25.

36 Zilberman Y, Cohen, B, Becker A. Familial trends in palatal canines, anomalous lateral incisors, and related phenomena. *Eur J Orthod* 1990; **12**: 135–139.

37 Takahama Y, Akiyama Y. Maxillary canine impaction as a possible microform of cleft lip and palate. *Eur J Orthod* 1982; **4**: 275–277.

38 Ericson S, Kürol J. Early treatment of palatally erupting maxillary canines by extraction of the primary canines. *Eur J Orthod* 1988; **10**: 283–295.

39 Power SM, Short MBE. An investigation into the response of palatally displaced canines to the removal of deciduous canines and an assessment of factors contributing to favourable eruption. *Br J Orthod* 1993; **20**: 215–223.

40 Gregg TA. Surgical division and pulpotomy of a double incisor tooth. *Br Dent J* 1985; **159**: 254–255.

41 Adams CP. Relation of spacing of the upper central incisors to abnormal fraenum labii and other features of the dento-facial complex. *Dent Record* 1954; **74**: 72–86.

42 Popovich F, Thompson GW, Main PA. The maxillary interincisal diastema and its relationship to the superior labial frenum and intermaxillary suture. *Angle Orthod* 1977; **47**: 265–271.

43 Ferguson MWJ, Rix C. Pathogenesis of abnormal midline spacing of human central incisors. A histological study of the involvement of the labial frenum. *Br Dent J* 1983; **154**: 212–218.

44 Bergström K, Jensen R, Mörtensson B. The effect of superior labial frenectomy in cases with midline diastema. *Am J Orthod* 1973; **63**: 633–638.

45 Richardson A, Ana JR. Occlusion and malocclusion in Lagos. *J Dent* 1973; **1**: 134–139.

46 Bowden BD. A longitudinal study of digital and dummy sucking. *Aust Dent J* 1966; **11**: 184–190.

47 Ruttle AT. et al. A serial study of the effects of finger-sucking. *J Dent Res* 1953; **32**: 739–748.

48 Leighton BC. The early signs of malocclusion. *Eur Orthod Soc Trans* 1969: 353–368.

49 Levine RS. Briefing paper: oral aspects of dummy and digit sucking. *Br Dent J* 1999; **186**: 108.

50 Subtelny JD, Subtelny JD. Oral habits - studies in form, function and therapy. *Angle Orthod* 1973; **43**: 347–383.

51 Barnett DP. An unusual transposition. *Br J Orthod* 1977; **4**: 149.

52 Avramaki E, Stephens CD. The effect of balanced and unbalanced extraction of primary molars on the relationship of incisor centrelines - a pilot study. *J Paed Dent* 1988; **4**: 9–12.

Summary of evidence for Chapter 8

Topic	Findings	Author/s
Relationship between local factors	69–79% had solitary anomaly, 18–28% had 1 additional disturbance, 2–3% had 2 additional disturbances. Hypothesis: common, possibly hereditary, aetiology with incomplete penetrance. Ectopic canines had high prevalence in all other groups.	Bjerklin et al 1992.[2] Clinical and radiographic study of 92 with first molar impaction, 93 with submerged molars, 91 with ectopic canines, 97 with absence of premolars.
Missing teeth	Excluding third molars, 3.3% had missing teeth. One or more third molar absent in 18.9%. Order of frequency: lower 5, upper 2, upper 5, lower 1, upper 4, lower 2. Lower 5 more frequently missing on left side.	Davies 1968.[3] Crossectional study of 950F, 1220M age 14 in Sydney. X-rays for 8s in 297F,374M
Association between agenesis, crowding and jaw relationship	Crowding in buccal segments less common in agenesis. Skeletal Class I and skeletal deep bite more common in agenesis group.	Dermaut et al 1986.[4] Cephalometric comparison of 185 with agenesis, including clefts, and controls. Sassouni analysis
Early extraction of E when 5 is missing	4 yrs after extraction, residual space in lower =2mm and in upper <1mm. Rate of space closure not related to age. Late extraction followed by tipping of adjacent teeth.	Lindqvist 1980.[6] Serial cast and x-ray study of 101 age 5–12yrs who had extraction of E and absence of 5.

Outcome of autotransplanting premolars

	Root formation at transplantation		Andreasen et al 1990.[8]
	Incomplete	**Complete**	Longitudinal study of 370 auto-
Survival	95%	98%	transplanted premolars over
Pulp healing	96%	15%	1–13yrs.
Root resorption		increase ⟶	
Final root length		increase ⟶	

Size of apical foramen and aseptic technique improved pulp healing. Initial ectopic position of graft and damage to Hertwig's sheath related to reduced root growth.

Dental anomalies of number, form and size

In the deciduous dentition each anomaly occurred in less than 1% excepting double teeth (1.6%).

Brook 1974.[9] Clinical and x-ray exam. of 611 age 3–5yrs and 1,115 age 11–14yrs British children in Slough

Prevalence at age 11–14 years.

	F	M	Total
Supernumeraries	1.7%	2.4%	2.1%
Hypodontia	5.7%	3.1%	4.4%
Invagination	2.4%	5.3%	4.1%
Double teeth			0.1%
Megadontia	0.9%	1.2%	1.1%
Microdontia	3.1%	1.9%	2.5%

Topic	Findings	Author/s
Effects of premaxillary super numeraries	Conical, incisiform, higher & smaller types with well-developed roots associated with eruption of incisors. Larger, lower, tuberculate, vertical & odontome types having poor roots associated with delayed eruption.	De Biase 1969.[10] Casts, X-rays and extracted teeth of 165 patients with premaxillary supernumeraries
Eruption to occlusion after exposure	11 teeth erupted at 1–2mm/month with reduction until occlusion at 90 months. 11 showed variations. Straight roots and open apices aided eruption. Crowding and soft tissues can delay eruption. Gingival level matches other side after 3 –10yrs. Maintaining exposure favours eruption.	Burke 1963.[11] Serial cast study of 22 incisor teeth after exposure
Emergence after supernumerary removal	78% erupted after median of 16 months. Where eruption failed, subsequent exposure was followed by eruption after a total of 30 months.	Mitchell, Bennett 1992.[15] Retrospective study of 120 incisors after removal of supernumerary teeth
Premature loss and eruption of successors	The earlier the loss, the earlier the eruption except lower premolars. Pattern is modified by space loss and delayed development. Premature loss of lower C delays eruption of 3.	Kerr 1980.[19] Longitudinal cast study of 126 subjects from 5–15yrs
Submerged deciduous molars	All submerged teeth were ankylosed. Presence of successors associated with diminished submergence but not with root resorption or bone growth at alveolar crest. Direct osteoid deposition in resorption lacunae. Opinion: early extraction of submerged molars prevents premolar open bite.	Rygh & Reitan 1963.[21] Cast, radiography and histology of 71 submerged teeth in 14F,17M
Submerged deciduous molars	All submerged deciduous molars shed within normal time. Normal bone heights resulted on both sides. Space loss on extraction side, occasionally serious.	Kürol & Koch 1985.[22] Prospective comparison of extraction/non extraction in homologous pairs of teeth.
Submerged primary molars	All except 5 submerged molars exfoliated with delay of about 6 months. Negative effects on occlusion usually temporary. Extraction required in severe infraocclusion and tipping of adjacent teeth and malposed successor.	Kürol & Thilander 1984.[23] Longitudinal cast and x-ray study of 149 submerged molars in 56 children until exfoliation
Age and overjet in relation to traumatised incisors	Frequency of traumatised incisors 6.5 times (F) and 5.0 times (M) higher in extreme vs normal overjet. Estimated that 50% of girls and more than 70% of boys received injuries before age 10yrs. Early treatment of extreme overjet recommended where possible.	Järvinen 1979.[25] Retrospective study of 716F,721M. Overjets classified Normal, increased, extreme. Age groups 7–9, 10–12, 13–16yrs

Topic (continued)	Findings	Author/s
Lower arch crowding	Increasing crowding related to forward movement of first molars. Lower incisors proclined.	Richardson ME 1979.[28] Longitudinal study of 51 children with third molars at ages 13 and 18yrs.
Effect of extraction of teeth on third molar development	Third molar impactions: non-extraction 34% first premolar extractions 28% second premolar extractions 17% molar extractions 0%	Richardson ME 1975.[29] Longitudinal cast and cephalometric study of 315 lower third molars with extraction of other teeth from 9yrs to eruption.
Effect of second molar extraction on third molar eruption	All third molars erupted from 3-10yrs after second molar extraction. 96% erupted in good or acceptable positions. 99% uprighted mesio-distally but few became as upright as the second molar they replaced	Richardson ME & Richardson 1993.[30] Longitudinal cast and cephalometric study of third molar eruption in 63 with second molar extraction.
Normal maxillary canine eruption	Unusual orientation of radiographs. Posterior movement 7-13yrs, vertical movement 5-13yrs. Palatal movement up to two years before eruption, buccal movement thereafter. Total movement 22mm.	Coulter & Richardson 1997.[33] Longitudinal study of normal canine eruption in 15F,15M in three dimensions from 5-15yrs.
Ectopic maxillary canine eruption	Compared with normal, ectopic teeth showed more anterior movement 7-12yrs, diminished vertical movement 6-13yrs. Consistent palatal movement at all ages.	McSherry & Richardson 1999.[34] Longitudinal study of ectopic canine eruption (20 teeth) in three dimensions from 5–15yrs.
Palatal canines related to dental anomalies in families of the propositi and 18 siblings.	Prevalence: **Popul.** **Parents** **Siblings** Palatal canine 1.5% 5.1% 11.4% Anomalies lateral 7.1% 30.8% 28.0% Delayed dental development in 2 of the propositi and 18 siblings.	Zilberman et al 1990.[36] Parents and siblings of 8F,17M with palatal canines examined for ectopic canines, dental development and anomalous lateral incisors.
Impacted canine as possible micro-fom of cleft lip and palate	Impacted canine in 0.74% of cleft parents and 0.27% of non-cleft. In cleft group, all impaction in fathers of cleft lip and palate children. None in other varieties of clefting. In control group, both parents involved.	Takahama & Akiyama 1982.[37] Prevalence of impacted upper canine in 408 parents of cleft children and 2959 parents of non-cleft children compared.
Early treatment of palatal canines by extraction of primary canines	78% of canines changed from palatal position to normal. If overlap less than ½ lateral root, 91% normalised, if more than ½, 64% normalised. In 8 of the 10 not improving, overlap was more than breadth of lateral root. No new improvements after 12 months.	Ericson & Kürol 1988.[38] Prospective extraction of primary canine in 35 consecutive subjects age 10–13yrs with 46 ectopic canines. X-ray follow-up for 18 months.
Relation between fraenum and diastema	In spaced arches fraenum determines the site of spacing. Size of fraenum unimportant. May interrupt transseptal fibres.	Adams 1954.[41]
Relation between fraenum, inter-maxillary suture and diastema	Fraena and suture types are related. Suture type remains constant. In some, fraena attachment rises. 159 of 230 diastemata closed by 16yrs. Minor contribution of fraena and sutures to diastema.	Popovich et al 1977.[42] Dental cast and cephalometric study of 471 at 9 and 16yrs and 230 annually who had diastema.
The fraenum and transseptal fibres	Fraenal fibres inhibit transseptal fibre formation.	Ferguson & Rix 1983.[43] Histology of 3 cadavera.
Effect of fraenectomy on midline diastema	Significant differences in closure of diastema at 6 months, 2 and 5yrs. Differences at 10yrs not significant. Diastema completely closed in 18 of 20 with fraenectomy and in 13 of 17 controls. Diastema may close spontaneously as late as 14-19yrs	Bergström et al 1973.[44] Prospective randomised study of fraenectomy results over 10yrs in 20 with 17 controls. None had very hyperplastic fraenum.
Dummy and digit sucking	Non-nutritional sucking in 80%. All dummy suckers ceased by 2.5 yrs. 21 of 45 digit suckers persisted to 8yrs. Nagging, gloves, bitter aloes and substitution of dummy for digit had limited success.	Bowden 1966.[46] Serial study of 58F,58M from 2–8yrs and questionnaires.
Thumb and finger sucking	Proclination and spacing of upper incisors. Rare increase in maxillary inter-canine width. Little effect on molar width in either arch.	Ruttle et al 1953.[47] Longitudinal cast study of 36 children with habits from about 4 to teenage.
Tongue thrusting	Tongue movements in swallowing adapted to variations in anterior malocclusion. Effect of tongue crib only temporary. Myofunctional therapy did not change basic protrusion pattern. Tongue function improved following orthodontic or surgical treatment	Subtelny & Subtelny 1973.[50] Report several studies at Eastman (New York) involving cineradiography.
Balanced and unbalanced loss of primary molars	1 Mean shift with no loss = 0.97mm 2 With balanced loss = 0.86mm 3 With unbalanced loss = 1.69mm Differences between means less than 1mm but statistically significant differences between 1 and 3 and 2 and 3.	Avramaki & Stephens 1988.[52] Cast study of midline shift in 19 with no loss, 15 balanced and 24 unbalanced loss. 21 of the 24 had loss of Es.

Patient examination for interception

While the following recommendations for patient examination are related to the ages of special vigilance described in Chapter 2, it should be kept in mind that patients vary in the timing of their development. Ideally, these ages of special vigilance should be related to the stage of dental development rather than to chronological age, but large differences between chronological age and dental stage may be significant in themselves and it is unreasonable to expect untrained people such as parents or headmasters to arrange for examination at specific dental stages. With this reservation, the ages will be found appropriate for the majority of Caucasian children. They may need adjustment in parts of the world where teeth erupt earlier or later.

It should be emphasised that the system of examination described in this chapter is specifically to identify patients suitable for interceptive treatment and does not replace the routine medical and dental history. It brings together the yardstick of normal eruption and occlusal development described in Chapter 2, the radiological stages of development in Chapter 3, the skeletal relationships and facial growth in Chapter 4, maturation of the soft tissues in Chapter 5, the possibilities for early interceptive treatment in Chapter 6 and the treatment of space deficiency and local irregularities in Chapters 7 and 8 respectively.

Standard examination

The standard clinical examination should include the following:

- Skeletal relationships: axial inclination of incisors, the profile.
- Soft tissues: lip competence at rest, tongue function at rest, during swallowing and speech, the periodontal condition.
- Tooth identification: absences or excesses, abnormalities of form or calcification, caries.
- Space conditions.
- Local abnormalities.
- Occlusion: buccal segment relationship, overjet and overbite, the relationship of the midlines to each other and to the middle of the face.
- Displacement of the mandible in closing from the rest position, dysfunction of the temporo-mandibular joint and muscles of mastication.

Screening at age 3 years

Skeletal discrepancies: at age 3 years these are best left untreated until a later stage.

Soft tissue abnormalities: abnormalities such as lisping and a tooth-apart swallow are common and likely to improve spontaneously.

Tooth identification: at age 3 years one expects to find a fully developed deciduous dentition. If there are abnormalities beyond the 95% limit, the stage of development may be compared with radiological standards.

Space conditions: spaces between the deciduous incisors and anthropoid spaces are normal and beneficial in accommodating the permanent teeth. Parents may need reassurance on this point. If there are no spaces in the deciduous dentition, crowding of the permanent teeth is predictable.

Local irregularities: absence of deciduous teeth is unusual. When it occurs, absence of the corresponding permanent tooth will almost certainly follow.

Supernumerary teeth are rare in the deciduous dentition. When they occur, there may be a corresponding supernumerary tooth in the permanent dentition.

Early loss of deciduous teeth at age 3 years is a serious matter. The most common cause is feeding-bottle caries, and parents should be advised appropriately.

Gemination between two deciduous incisors is usually followed by absence of a permanent tooth. Gemination between a deciduous incisor and a supernumerary element may be followed by a supernumerary permanent tooth, a permanent tooth of abnormal form or there may be no abnormality.

A large labial fraenum with a low attachment is not abnormal at this stage, and upper midline diastema is common.

Habits such as thumbsucking are frequent. The attention of the parent should be drawn to the possible effects on the permanent dentition if the habit is persistent.

Occlusion: having the distal surfaces of the second molars in the same vertical plane is the rule rather than the exception. A substantially increased overbite and overjet of the deciduous incisors suggest that there will be a similar relationship in the permanent dentition.

Displacements: of the mandible, in closing from the rest position, should be treated early so that occlusal development may proceed on the basis of an undisplaced jaw relationship. Plans should be made to treat displacements by grinding or extraction of deciduous canines or by expansion of the deciduous arch if severe crossbites exist.

Pathological lesions such as apical abscesses should always be sought and treated.

Screening at age 7–9 years

Skeletal discrepancies: are not normally treated at this age, but plans can be made to use a functional appliance during the puberal growth spurt.

Soft tissue abnormalities: abnormalities such as lisping are common and have a good prospect for spontaneous improvement.

Tooth identification: the first permanent molars should have erupted and the permanent incisors should be erupting. Delayed eruption of a tooth beyond the 95% limits given in Chapter 2 merits radiological investigation. This is a good time to make a radiological review of the developing dentition. The stage of development should be compared with the illustrations in Chapter 3.

Space conditions: crowding of the incisors when they first erupt in Caucasian children is the rule rather than the exception. At the lower end of this age range, there is still the prospect of slight improvement by lateral jaw growth and spontaneous proclination. Where crowding is minimal, effective use of the leeway space by fitting a lingual arch may be sufficient. Should the crowding be greater, serial extraction may be appropriate. If the deciduous canines and molars are still present, the likelihood is that there will be sufficient space to accommodate their permanent successors.

If the first permanent molars are grossly carious or hypoplastic their extraction should be considered.

Local irregularities: absence of lower central or upper lateral incisors may be noted. If an upper lateral incisor is absent, eruption of the corresponding canine may be delayed. The upper end of this age range is a good time to extract second deciduous molars where the second premolars are absent.

Should a single deciduous molar need to be extracted, space maintenance is the best option in normally developing occlusions. If this is contraindicated, compensating and balancing extractions may be needed in the case of first deciduous molars.

Prolonged retention of deciduous incisors should be treated by extraction if they are displacing the permanent incisors.

If eruption of an upper incisor is delayed beyond the 95% limit or if it is severely rotated, the presence of a supernumerary tooth is always a possibility. Early extraction of the supernumerary tooth is indicated.

Supplemental incisors are usually treated by extraction.

Teeth of abnormal form should be noted. Small upper lateral incisors may be associated with invagination or impending delay in the eruption of the maxillary canines.

Abnormal fraena should be noted but not necessarily treated at this stage.

There may be an upper midline diastema and fanning of upper incisors at this ugly duckling stage. The presence of a supernumerary tooth may be suspected if there is a large and persistent upper midline diastema. Radiographic examination should not be delayed. Quite substantial spontaneous closure of the diastema may occur following extraction of the supernumerary tooth.

Habits should be discouraged. A deterrent appliance may be helpful.

If the permanent canines are not palpable at the end of this age range, the patient should be monitored carefully with the prospect of extracting both upper deciduous canines. Extraction of transposed lower lateral incisors should be considered.

Impaction of upper first permanent molars should be observed or treated depending on severity. There is little prospect of spontaneous resolution after age 8 years.

Occlusion: there is frequently a transitional open bite which will be corrected spontaneously. The antero-posterior occlusion of the first permanent molars may be slightly post-normal with the prospect of spontaneous correction. Attrition of the remaining deciduous teeth is generally a favourable sign. This is a good time to procline upper incisors in lingual occlusion where the dental base relationship is skeletal I or a mild skeletal III. The upper removable appliance may be supplemented with a chincap if there is a moderate Class III skeletal pattern.

Displacements: of the mandible, in closing from the rest position, should be treated early so that occlusal development may proceed on the basis of an undisplaced jaw relationship. Proclination of upper incisors in cases of lingual occlusion will deal with any anterior displacement. Minor unilateral crossbites with displacements of the mandible may improve when habits are abandoned and the deciduous canines are shed. More prominent displacements should be treated by grinding or extraction of deciduous canines or by expansion of the upper arch.

Screening at age 11–12 years

Skeletal discrepancies: may be treated with a functional appliance in females but may be delayed for a year in males.

Soft tissue abnormalities: the behaviour of the soft tissues should have matured.

Tooth identification: the premolars, second molars and canines should be erupting.

Space conditions: a canine and premolars of average size can usually be accommodated if the distance between the distal surface of the lateral incisor and the mesial surface of the first molar is 22mm or more. A mixed dentition analysis will give more accurate estimates.

This is the best time to treat crowding interceptively by extraction of premolars or to plan extraction of second molars.

Local irregularities: absence of an upper lateral incisor may be related to delayed eruption of the corresponding maxillary canine. Decide whether the canine should be brought down alongside the central incisor or whether it should be placed distally with artificial replacement of the lateral. Where second premolars are absent, it is too late to expect total spontaneous space closure following extraction of second deciduous molars in the lower jaw.

Supernumerary teeth in the upper midline causing rotation or delayed eruption of a central incisor or midline diastema should be removed immediately. Erupted supplemental teeth usually cause crowding and an extraction is indicated.

Early loss of deciduous teeth may have led to secondary crowding of premolars which may be treated by extraction or regaining the lost space.

Retained deciduous teeth which are deflecting their successors should be removed. Submerged deciduous molars should be kept under observation. If there is any apparent risk of them becoming completely submerged, they should be removed and space maintenance considered.

Impaction of second premolars should be treated by extraction of other teeth, by creating space for eruption with an appliance or by extraction of second premolars themselves.

Delayed eruption of a tooth beyond 95% limits merits radiological investigation.

Abnormally formed upper lateral incisors should be examined for invagination and the position of the corresponding canine investigated.

Abnormally large and fibrous upper fraena are often excised at this time. The associated diastema will tend to close spontaneously under the influence of the erupting canines and contraction of scar tissue.

Any transient upper midline diastema related to the ugly duckling stage should be closing with the prospect of further closure up to age 14 and beyond. If a large persistent diastema exists, urgent radiological investigation is needed.

Habits should be vigorously discouraged.

If the maxillary canines are not palpable in the buccal sulcus they should be investigated radiologically and treated by extraction of the deciduous canines.

The transposition most commonly detected at this stage is between the maxillary canine and first premolar. Interceptive treatment in the form of extraction of one of the transposed teeth may be appropriate if some space closure has occurred.

Occlusion: the first molars should be in normal occlusion if the deciduous molars have been shed. If the malocclusion is to be treated without premolar or first molar extraction, the upper first molars may be moved distally at this stage in Class II cases.

Transitional open bites should have closed.

Displacements: anterior displacements should be treated urgently by proclination of upper incisors and grinding or extraction of deciduous canines if they are still present. Lateral displacements with crossbites may be difficult to treat at this stage through lack of teeth.

The possibility of pathological conditions should be kept in mind.

Dos and don'ts

Some of the dos and don'ts of interceptive orthodontics are summarised in Table 9.1.

This system of examination, with radiography, is sufficiently detailed to support clinical decisions in most cases.

Kirschen[1] has proposed a more basic screening examination to identify those children who are likely to benefit from orthodontic care or referral to an orthodontist without specifying the form of treatment. The chief advantage of the Kirschen system is that the screening can be done in schools, in community clinics or by the busy practitioner in less than a minute. The screening at age 9 years consists of five clinical triggers for further investigation. These are:

- Delayed eruption as judged by an abnormal sequence or comparison with the contralateral side;
- Crowding as judged by overlapping teeth or lateral incisors almost in contact with first deciduous molars;
- Overjet which exceeds 4mm;
- Crossbites without assessing displacement at this stage;
- Submergence of deciduous molars.

Recommended additional triggers not included in the 60 second screening are:

- Caries with particular reference to carious or hypoplastic first molars or early loss of deciduous canines or molars;
- Deep overbite or open bite which are not included in the 1 minute examination because it is likely that they would be found in conjunction with another trigger.

A further additional trigger appropriate at age 12 years is:

- Palpation for unerupted canines.

Reference

Kirschen R. Orthodontic clinical screening in under a minute. *Br Dent J* 1998; **185**: 224–226.

Table 9.1 The dos and don'ts of interceptive orthodontics.

Do	Age	Don't
Encourage general and local caries prevention.	Birth	Worry about seemingly abnormal relationships of the gum pads.
Look for the early signs of malocclusion. Expect crowded permanent teeth if no spaces exist. Discourage habits. Treat abnormal closure path.	3yrs	Worry about lisping. Worry about spaced incisors or anthropoid spaces. Worry about distal surfaces of second deciduous molars in vertical line.
Investigate delayed eruption. Observe or use leeway space in minimal crowding. If crowding is greater, consider serial extraction or extraction of first molars if carious or hypoplastic. Maintain space if appropriate. Extract second deciduous molars if second premolars are absent. Extract retained deciduous and supernumerary teeth causing malocclusion. Strongly discourage habits. Observe or treat impacted upper first molars. Consider extraction of transposed teeth. Treat incisors in lingual occlusion. Treat pathology early.	7–9yrs	Worry about slight post-normality of first molars. Worry about midline diastema or 'ugly duckling' when incisors first erupt. Worry about slight anterior open bite.
Watch for crowding and consider first premolar or second molar extractions. Extract deciduous teeth deflecting permanent successors. Excise very large fraena where there is an upper midline diastema. Discourage habits vigorously. Extract upper deciduous canines when permanent canines are ectopically placed. Treat incisors in lingual occlusion urgently.	11–12yrs	Worry about buccal segment crowding if deciduous canine and molars present or if 22mm between distal of lateral and mesial of first molar. Worry about rotated premolars when they first erupt. Worry about minor submergence of deciduous molars.

10 Interception in context

Malocclusion may appear in the form of crowding or spacing of the teeth, local irregularities, abnormal relationship of the arches, abnormal relationship of the jaw bones or any of these in combination. The malocclusion may be accepted. It may be treated interceptively, with removable appliances, with functional appliances, with fixed appliances, with orthognathic surgery or with a combination of these treatment methods.

Acceptance

Accepting the malocclusion may be justified if the irregularity is slight, if it does not threaten dental health or masticatory efficiency, and if the patient can be persuaded to accept any cosmetic detriment. Any malocclusion may be accepted if the patient will not have treatment. Acceptance has no cost and carries no risk of iatrogenic change.

Interception

Interceptive treatment is inexpensive, has none of the risks of appliance therapy, and has no risk of relapse resulting from the teeth being placed in unstable positions. Interception is best suited to treatment of displacements, crowding and local irregularities. The timing of interceptive treatment is critical. The outcome may not meet high standards of tooth positioning and undesirable tooth movements may occur. Successful interceptive treatment needs knowledge and experience. The basic principle of interceptive orthodontics is to promote naturally occurring changes which are favourable and to suppress factors which lead to malposition of the teeth and malocclusion. In some cases, counselling is all that is required; in others, space maintenance, simple appliance therapy, extraction of teeth, modification of the shape of teeth or local surgical intervention may be appropriate.

Removable appliances

Removable appliances are inexpensive, facilitate mouth hygiene, are easy to repair and gain much anchorage from the palate and alveolar processes. Any risk of traumatic injury from distortion or breakage can be dealt with by the patient removing the appliance. Removable appliances tip teeth. They are unsuitable for elongations, rotations and apical or bodily movements unless combined with a fixed attachment on the tooth in question. Relative intrusion or extrusion of a group of teeth is possible using a bite plane. Abnormal relationships of the arches can be treated with removable appliances if there is no skeletal discrepancy. Transient inflammation of the mucosa often occurs under removable appliances.

Functional appliances

Functional appliances are inexpensive, carry little risk of damaging the teeth or gingivae and can be removed by the patient in an emergency. They are at their best in the treatment of abnormal relationships of the arches and may have beneficial effects in skeletal discrepancy cases. Functional appliances will not produce elongation, rotation or apical movement of individual teeth. They are best used during a growth spurt.

Fixed appliances

Fixed appliances can be used for elongation, rotation and apical or bodily movement of teeth. Very precise positioning of teeth is possible in skilled hands. They can be used to camouflage moderate skeletal discrepancies. Fixed appliance therapy is expensive and may be associated with decalcification, root resorption and some loss of crestal bone. Some fixed appliances are heavily dependent on extra-oral anchorage. Teeth may be moved readily into unstable positions. A degree of relapse following treatment is frequent.[1] Breakage of appliances needs early attention from the orthodontist.

Orthognathic surgery

Surgical treatment of skeletal discrepancies is almost invariably combined with fixed appliance therapy. The combination is the most versatile of treatments available. It is extremely expensive and has all the risks of fixed appliance therapy with additional surgical and anaesthetic risks.

Some of the advantages and disadvantages of these treatment methods are shown in Table 10.1

Orthodontics for the individual

The fashion in orthodontics today is for pre-programmed fixed appliances with average figures for tip, torque and in-out compensations built into each bracket. When the treatment goes according to plan, the result is visually very attractive indeed and a source of great joy to the

Table 10.1 Advantages and limitations of treatment methods.

Treatment	Advantages	Limitations
Acceptance	No cost, No risk	No change
Interception	Not expensive No risk of decalcification, root resorption or soft tissue problems	Timing critical May not be completely effective May allow undesirable changes Limited to displacements, crowding & local irregularities
Removable appliances	Inexpensive Little risk of decalcification or root resorption Inexpensive repairs Patient removes in emergency Good anchorage	Principally tipping movements No elongations, rotations, apical movements of individual teeth unless combined with fixed attachment Treat moderate skeletal problems by dental compensation
Functional appliances	Inexpensive Little risk of decalcification or root resorption Treat inter-arch discrepancies Treat skeletal problems	Little local effect No elongations, rotations or apical movements of individual teeth
Fixed appliances	Can elongate, rotate and move apices Excellent detailing Can camouflage skeletal discrepancies	Expensive Possible decalcification, root resorption, bone loss Anchorage problems Emergencies which need orthodontist Possible instability of results
Surgery	Decisive treatment of skeletal discrepancies	Expensive Surgical and anaesthetic risks Some instability

patient and the orthodontist. Most orthodontists with manual skill enjoy working with fixed appliances, can demand high fees and are seen to be keeping pace with modern developments. However, there is little evidence that teeth in these average positions are any more durable than those which are not and some relapse following treatment is frequent.[1] Not every treatment goes according to plan. If the appliance is fully worked out, the incisor teeth are left at average inclinations which may not be compatible with an average overjet when the skeletal pattern deviates from normal.

Such skeletal problems may be treated surgically or in a preliminary phase with a functional appliance during the period of active growth. The combination of surgery and fixed appliance therapy may be seen as the acme of skill but it is extremely expensive and carries a high risk of iatrogenic effects.

Removable appliances are an inexpensive and safe way of tipping teeth. To take the simplest example, labial movement of an upper incisor out of lingual occlusion can be best achieved with a removable appliance. Using a fixed appliance in the same situation is unnecessarily expensive and has the difficulty of gaining attachment to loosening deciduous molars. Although useful, removable appliances rarely act on all teeth simultaneously. Consequently, treatment goals are limited and there may be residual irregularities which adversely affect assessment ratings and changes in indices of treatment need.

If interception is taken to include early treatment with removable, functional appliances and the chincap, it offers a quite versatile system for young children without necessarily treating every malocclusion to completion. Interception must have a place in the armamentarium of every orthodontist. For example, it is not clever to delay treatment of palatally placed maxillary canines until ready for exposure followed by alignment with fixed appliances when the beneficial effects of deciduous canine extraction are well known.

The suitability of treatment methods in the various types of malocclusion is shown in Table 10.2.

Orthodontics in the community

Opinions vary on the best orthodontic service for a community.

Some would say that almost all malocclusions should be treated in the established dentition with fixed appliances and surgery if necessary. Unless the number of orthodontists and the attendant funding increases exponentially there seems little hope of satisfying the demand or need for orthodontic treatment with fixed appliances in the forseeable future. The imbalance between the supply and demand or need for orthodontic treatment could be met by restricting the demand or by making full use

Table 10.2 Suitability of treatment methods for malocclusions seen early and late

Malocclusion	Early	Late
Spacing		Removable or fixed appliance
Crowding	Intercept	Removable or fixed appliance
Local irregularities	Intercept	Removable or fixed appliance
Abnormal arch relationships	Functional or removable appliance	Removable or fixed appliance
Abnormal jaw relationships	Functional appliance chincap	Surgery

of simpler, less expensive treatments. Emphasis has been placed on limiting the demand by setting the need, which is determined by dentists and orthodontists, at a reasonably high level. Against the background of restricted public funds the question being asked is whether every malocclusion, however mild, should be treated. The consensus opinion is that patients with trivial irregularities should not qualify for treatment at public expense.

Many attempts have been made to devise indices which establish a cut off point in the scale of eligibility for treatment.[2–6] The most recent British proposal is the Index of Orthodontic Treatment Need devised by Brook and Shaw,[7] following the report of the Schanshieff Committee into unnecessary dental treatment.[8] Some problems with indices are that the scientific evidence of an association between malocclusion and dental disease is somewhat scant and that the index should be simple and comprehensible on the one hand and all embracing on the other. One factor which is difficult to define objectively and truthfully is the effect of the malocclusion on the morale of the individual patient.

The severity of the malocclusion is not necessarily related to the complexity and price of the appropriate appliance therapy. Given that public expenditure, rather than the malocclusion, is the primary factor in limiting the availability of orthodontic treatment, perhaps the real requirement is not for an index of treatment need but an index of treatment complexity or costs. At present, there is no index of complexity which is particularly satisfactory but as a crude interim measure, three grades of complexity based on the PAR index have been proposed.[9] Interceptive treatment which is very inexpensive might be made available to all patients where it will be beneficial. At the other end of the scale, any patient with severe occlusal problems in need of surgery should receive it without question. Patients in the intermediate grades of treatment complexity and expense might be placed on a scale depending on available resources. Rich authorities which place a high priority on orthodontic care might provide all classes of treatment; others with limited funding might provide removable and functional appliances but not fixed appliances. Some may limit orthodontic care to interception.

The present emphasis on fixed appliances in this country has ensured that orthodontists see interceptive orthodontics as unfashionable, anachronistic and contrary to the image they wish to project. Early detection has been handed down to the general practitioner by default. Although the general practitioner may be strategically placed to identify and treat developing malocclusions in the patients he sees, the chain of referral to a specialist or consultant in doubtful cases often results in the child being seen too late for effective interceptive treatment. In any event, 39% of children aged 8 years and 36% aged 12 years do not attend a practitioner regularly.[10] These deprived children have little chance of receiving interceptive treatment unless the anomaly is detected by a community dentist while screening for dental caries and the periodontal diseases. Estimates of the unmet need for orthodontic treatment in British children aged 14–16 years range from 20 to 34%.[10–13]

In the interceptive context, the unpublished work of Roberts[14] suggested that screening with a view to interception could be beneficial in small closed communities and Chung and Kerr,[15] without investigating the effectiveness of treatment, showed that young patients in Glasgow found interception an acceptable form of therapy.

Reports of the number of children whose dentitions would benefit from interception are difficult to evaluate and compare because of differing interpretations of where interceptive orthodontics begins and ends, differences between the range of treatments on offer, differences between aims and differences between the samples examined. Two long-term American studies have been carried out in Burlington[16] where 49% of the sample responded to interceptive treatment, and in Pennsylvania[17,18] where favourable responses were variously reported to be 14.3%[17] or 15–20%.[18] The latter publication under the title ' Preventive and interceptive orthodontics: a strong theory proves weak in practice' provoked a sharp response from Moyers,[19] who pointed out that the real world of appliance therapy is a tough, difficult game and if one in five children can be treated interceptively, this would make a very significant contribution to the treatment of malocclusion in the community. The British study conducted by Hiles[20] in Winchester revealed that 38.6% of her sample would benefit from interception.

At first reading, the large disparity between these figures is remarkable until one realises, for example, that the objective in Burlington[16] was to reduce or eliminate malocclusion (18% without appliances, 31% with appliances) whereas in Pennsylvania[17,18] the aim was to eliminate malocclusion so that there was no need for further treatment. In the Winchester study, Hiles[20] permitted simple appliance therapy with the aim of reducing or eliminating malocclusion. The similarities and contrasts between these four studies are shown in Table 10.3

The fact that there are ages of special vigilance for interception has led to the proposal that the child population should be screened at these ages and interceptive measures applied where appropriate. There is a strong case for taking interception into the community as a screening procedure, but it is vitally important that those conducting the screening are made fully aware of what it is they are trying to do. The traditional screening for malocclusion always produces figures for treatment need which vary between one observer and another and simply confirm the known fact that the combined need and demand exceeds the available manpower. Such surveys may be counterproductive in that they may stimulate a demand which cannot be met at present.

What is required is a screening procedure specifically and exclusively to identify and offer treatment to those children who would benefit from interceptive orthodontics. Some radiology would be essential in such an exercise but the balance between the risks and benefits in radiography demand that radiological examination should be preceded by clinical examination and consent.

There can be little doubt of the cost-effectiveness of such a scheme. Taking one small facet alone, the extraction of deciduous canines to redirect eruption of ectopic maxillary canines would save sufficient surgical and orthodontic time to justify the project. The alternative, involving exposure of the canine (often under general anaesthesia) followed by orthodontic alignment is very expensive. National Health Service costings for this type of treatment do not seem to exist, but there is no doubt that it can be reckoned in millions of pounds annually. It is also significant that previous reports of long-term interceptive studies[16–18,20] predate the Ericson and Kürol work on interception of maxillary canine impaction.[21] Similarities and differences between the present and previous definitions of interceptive treatment are shown in Table 10.4.

Table 10.3 Similarities and contrasts between previous community studies.

	Burlington[16]	**Pennsylvania**[17,18]	**Winchester**[20]
Sample	312	4,200	1,837
Origin	Community	Self-selecting	Community
Age	3–6, 6–9, 9–12, 12–16 years	1,445 in primary or mixed dentition	9+ years
Exclusions	Appliance therapy	Extraction of permanent teeth, space maintenance or regaining, skeletal problems	Class II malocclusion
Aim	Reduce or eliminate malocclusion	Eliminate malocclusion	Reduce or eliminate malocclusion
Benefiting	49%	15%	38.6%

Table 10.4 Similarities and differences between previous and present definitions of interceptive treatment.

	Burlington[16]	Pennsylvania[17,18]	Winchester[20]	Richardson
Extraction of deciduous teeth	Yes	Yes	Yes	Yes
Extraction of permanent teeth	Yes	No	Yes	Yes
Space maintenance or regaining	Yes	No	No	Yes
Anterior open bite/habit	Yes	Yes	No	Yes
Increased overjet with spacing	No	Yes	No	Yes
Anterior displacement	No	Yes	Yes	Yes
Other displacement	No	Yes	No	Yes
Local factors	Yes	Yes	Yes	Yes

References

1　Little RM, Wallen TR, Reidel RA. Stability and relapse of mandibular anterior alignment - first premolar extraction cases treated by traditional edgewise orthodontics. *Am J Orthod* 1981; **80**: 349–365.

2　Grainger RM. *Orthodontic treatment priority index* PHS publication No.1000 Series 2 No.25 Washington: US. Government Printing Office. 1967.

3　Salzmann JA. A handicapping malocclusion assessment to establish treatment priority. *Am J Orthod* 1968; **54**: 749–765.

4　Summers CJ. The occlusal index. A system for identifying and scoring occlusal disorders. *Am J Orthod* 1971; **59**: 552–567.

5　Lundstrom A. Need for treatment in cases of malocclusion. *Eur Orthod Soc Trans* 1977: 111–123.

6　Linder-Aronson S. Orthodontics in the Swedish public dental health service. *Eur Orthod Soc Trans* 1974: 233–240.

7　Brook PH, Shaw WC. The development of an index of orthodontic treatment priority. *Eur J Orthod* 1989: **11**: 309–320.

8　Schanshieff SG. Report of the Committee of Enquiry into unnecessary Dental Treatment. London: HMSO: 1986.

9　Richmond S, Daniels CP, Wright J. The professional perception of orthodontic treatment complexity. *Br Dent J* 1997; **183**: 371–375.

10　O'Brien M. *Children's dental health in the United Kingdom.* Office of Publication Censuses and Surveys, Social Surveys Division: London, 1993.

11　Crabb JJ, Rock WP. Orthodontic screening of nine-year-old children. *Br J Orthod* 1986; **13**: 43–48.

12　Roberts E, Beales J, Dixon L, Willcocks A. The orthodontic condition and treatment status of a sample of 14-year-old children in North Derbyshire. *Comm Dent Health* 1989; **6**: 249–250.

13　Burden DJ, Mitropoulos CM, Shaw WC. Residual orthodontic need in a sample of 15- and 16- year- olds. *Br Dent J* 1994; **176**: 220–224.

14　Roberts GH. A manual of orthodontic screening for the use of the dental staff of the United States Navy at Royal Air Force Edzell, Scotland. Personal communication 1976.

15　Chung CK, Kerr WJS. Interceptive orthodontics: application and outcome in a demand population. *Br Dent J* 1987; **162**: 73–76.

16　Popovich F, Thompson GW. Evaluation of preventive and interceptive orthodontic treatment between 3 and 18 years of age. *Trans Third Int Cong Orthod* 1975: 260–281.

17　Freeman ID. Preventive and interceptive orthodontics: a critical review and the results of a clinical study. *J Prev Dent* 1977; **4**: 7–23.

18　Ackerman JL, Proffit WR. Preventive and interceptive orthodontics: a strong theory proves weak in practice. *Angle Orthod* 1980; **50**: 75–87.

19　Moyers RE. Editorial comment. *Yearbook of dentistry* Chicago: Yearbook Publishers, 1980: 3–39.

20　Hiles AM. Is orthodontic screening of 9-year-old children cost effective? *Br Dent J* 1985; **159**: 41–45.

21　Ericson S, Kürol J. Early treatment of palatally erupting maxillary canines by extraction of the primary canines. *Eur J Orthod* 1988; **10**: 283–295.

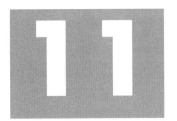

11 Community interception

While interception for the individual patient may be carried out in general practice, it is argued in Chapter 10 that if interception is to make any impact in meeting the need for orthodontic treatment it would be best practised in the environment of community dentistry. For the reasons given in Chapter 10, existing reports of interceptive projects conflict in their assessment of how large this impact would be. Accordingly, it was decided to validate the concept of interception described in this book in the Northern Ireland community.

The possibilities for interception seemed to be applicable at two dental stages – an early stage on eruption of the incisor teeth which has been loosely labelled 7–9 years and a later stage, primarily to identify ectopic canine teeth. The ages of eruption in the Belfast Growth Study material[1] indicated that 95% of upper lateral incisors had not erupted before 9.49 years in females and 9.77 years in males.[2] Work on the same material had shown that a substantial proportion of normally erupting maxillary canines had not made enough of their buccal movement to render them palpable in the buccal sulcus before 11 years.[3] Accordingly, the possibilities for interception were divided into those appropriate at 9 years and at 11 years. These are listed in Tables 11.1 and 11.2 respectively.

Since we were anxious not to over-treat or to over-state the case for interception, it was important to establish diagnostic cut-off points for quantifiable features of the developing occlusion which may correct spontaneously without any treatment whatever. Secondly, we needed to determine the reproducibility of diagnostic and treatment decisions. These were explored in a preliminary investigation on the Growth Study material which has been reported in detail elsewhere.[4]

Diagnostic cut-off points

The smallest distance between the distal surface of the permanent lateral incisor and mesial surface of the first permanent molar at age 9 years which was compatible with good alignment of the canine and premolar teeth after they had erupted was 18.75mm in the lower arch and 18.25mm in the upper arch. These were rounded into a common measurement of 18.5mm. The largest diastema between the upper central incisors at age 9 years which closed spontaneously was 2.50mm and the largest amount of crowding of the lower incisors at age 9 years which resolved spontaneously was 3.80mm.[5]

These measurements, together with a 6mm indent suitable for measuring overjets, were incorporated into a disposable plastic gauge, shown in Figure 11.1. The diastema measurement is at the top of the gauge, the lateral incisor-first molar measurement between the two peaks at the lower right and the 6mm overjet measurement between the right edge of the gauge and the first of the peaks. The left end of the gauge is stepped corresponding to 0.5mm, 1.0mm, 1.5mm and 2.0mm to facilitate measurement of lower incisor crowding. The overjet measurement was included because Järvinen[6,7] has shown that overjets beyond this figure increase the risk of traumatic injury to the upper incisors.

With the assistance of the gauge, all available casts of children in the Growth Study at the ages

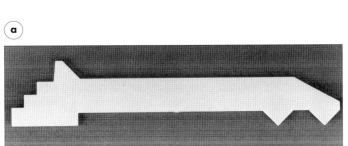

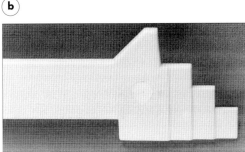

Fig. 11.1 The interception gauge. (a) the diastema measurement is at the top of the gauge, the lateral incisor-first molar measurement between the two peaks at the lower right and the 6mm measurement between the right end of the gauge and the first of the peaks. (b) the right end of the gauge has thicknesses corresponding to 0.5, 1.0, 1.5 and 2.0mm to facilitate measurement of incisor crowding.

Table 11.1 Interceptive possibilities at age 9 years.

Diagnosis	Treatment
Crowding	Distalise molar, extract incisor, premolar, first molar, serial extraction
Carious permanent first molar	Extract (? balance, compensate, appliance)
Delayed eruption	Investigate
Absent teeth	Close or maintain space
Recent extraction	Maintain space
Retained deciduous teeth	Extract
Unilateral retained deciduous canine	Extract
Erupted supernumerary tooth	Extract
Malformed teeth	Mask, extract, split
Local spacing	Remove pathology
Anterior open bite	Advise, deterrent appliance
Transposition	Extract
Molar impaction	Extract E, distalise, observe
Incisor in lingual occlusion (anterior displacement)	Procline
Lateral displacement	Grind or extract deciduous canines, expand
Increased overjet	Reduce overjet

Table 11.2 Interceptive possibilities at age 11 years.

Diagnosis	Treatment
Crowding	Distalise molar, extract incisor, premolar, first molar, second molar
Carious permanent first molar	Extract (? balance, compensate, appliance)
Delayed eruption	Investigate
Absent teeth	Close or maintain space
Erupted Supernumerary tooth	Extract
Retained deciduous teeth	Extract, observe submerged deciduous molars
Malformed teeth	Mask, extract, split
Local spacing	Remove pathology
Palpate for permanent canine	Extract deciduous canines
Incisor in lingual occlusion (anterior displacement)	Procline
Displacement	Grind or extract deciduous canines, expand

of 9 years ± 3 months (278 subjects) and 11 years ± 3 months (272 subjects) were screened independently by two investigators for the interceptive possibilities listed in Tables 11.1 and 11.2.

Reproducibility of assessments

The majority of treatment decisions were highly reproducible as tested by the Kappa statistic.[8] For the diagnostic categories the Kappa values were generally much more favourable than 0.8 which indicates good agreement between observers. In the treatment categories, the reproducibility of observations was also good or substantial (above 0.6).

Community study

The following is an overview of the community study which is reported in detail elsewhere.[9]

The purpose of the investigation was to explore the feasibility of incorporating screening for interception in routine community dental inspections, to make recommendations for treatment and to assess the outcome. For this purpose, large numbers of the interception gauge were produced in plastic disposable form by Messrs. Belmark Plastics*. The treatment goal was to reduce or eliminate malocclusion by any interceptive means, including simple removable appliance therapy as defined in this book. Only removable appliance treatment such as could be undertaken by a general practitioner trained in the Belfast school was allowed.

Subjects: the subjects were 2002 children who were to be screened in routine community dental inspections. There were 1002 children age 9 years ± 3 months and 1000 aged 11 years ± 3 months. Of the 2002 children, 1060 lived in the urban area of greater Belfast and 942 in the rural area of Enniskillen and Omagh, Co. Tyrone.

A form of consent was sent to the parents or guardians of all children explaining the nature of the investigation and asking for consent to examine the children at the time of the community dental inspection.

Those children found suitable for interception were sent an appointment to attend a local hospital accompanied by a responsible person. At the hospital visit, the precise nature of the malocclusion and proposed treatment was explained and impressions and radiographs (where required) were taken.

A letter was then sent to the general practitioner or community dentist asking for treatment to be carried out. Approximately 12 months later, the children and their parents were recalled to the local hospital for further impressions to record progress.

Integration with community dental inspections: with experience and the aid of the interception gauge, the screening time was reduced to approximately 2 minutes and integration with community dental inspections was achieved without difficulty.

Compliance: overall, consent to the initial examination was given for 90% of the children of whom 91% were present on the day of initial screening with the Community Dental Inspection. Interception was found to be appropriate for 33% of the children. Of those, only 62% kept the first hospital appointment. Only 62% of those attended on recall 12 months later, and of those only 71% had actually received the treatment requested.

Consent to the initial examination was about 10% higher and the percentage of those completing the full programme of visits was 14% higher in the rural as against the urban area. These differences were probably due to the greater availability of orthodontic care in the urban area but there was an almost equal reluctance on the part of urban and rural children or parents to fulfil the initial hospital visit. Overall, consent and compliance were disappointing. This calls into question the viability of any community interception scheme. It seems clear that some effort to promote the scheme among dentists and the general public would be required before it could make an appreciable contribution to solving the orthodontic manpower problem. However, two points may be made in mitigation. First, interception is particularly applicable in children with neglected mouths in terms of untreated displacements, retained roots of deciduous teeth, carious first molars etc. Thus, there would be a high proportion of children who are resistant to any form of dentistry in the interception groups. Secondly, we are unable to say whether children who failed the recall hospital appointment had the treatment implemented or not. It is possible that some children who received successful interceptive treatment may have been satisfied by the outcome but not sufficiently motivated by the research aspect of the project to keep the recall hospital appointment.

Malocclusions: of the children aged 9 years suitable for interception, the greatest need was for treatment of crowding (30%) followed by extraction of retained deciduous teeth (18%), unilateral retained deciduous canine (17%), displacement (15%), incisor in lingual occlusion (11%), increased overjet (10%) and carious permanent molar (6%). In the children aged 11 years suitable for interception, the greatest need was for treatment of crowding (45%) followed by retained deciduous teeth (28%), ectopic canine (12%), displacement (11%), carious molar (9%) and lingual occlusion (8%). It was not surprising to find that the greatest need was for treatment of crowding but the prevalence of ectopic maxillary canine at 12% was interesting in view of the efficacy of interceptive extraction of the deciduous canine in treating this condition.[10]

The expectation that there might be a greater need for interception in the rural area was not borne out by the findings. In fact the figures for those in need were 28% and 30% in Enniskillen at 9 and 11 years with corresponding figures of 34% and 38% in Belfast.

At both ages, there were significantly more carious first molars in Belfast with a higher percentage of retained deciduous teeth in Enniskillen/Omagh. At age 11 years, there was a higher percentage of displacements in the Enniskillen/Omagh area. None of the other differences exceeded 3%.

Treatment: only 104 children completed the full programme of attendance and had the treatment carried out. The treatment was extraction of deciduous teeth in 41%, extraction of permanent teeth in 33%, extraction of both deciduous and permanent teeth in 9%, appliance therapy in 12%, extractions with appliance therapy in 5% and fraenectomy in 1% of cases.

Outcome measures: outcomes were measured on casts from impressions at the first and final hospital visits in two ways. First, the dental health component of the Index of Orthodontic Treatment Need[11] was used, not so much to assess progress, but to determine the numbers of children in need of treatment at the beginning of the study and those in need of further treatment at the end. Secondly, local indices specific to the study were applied since IOTN scores only the most significant feature of the malocclusion (e.g. the overjet) which may not have been the irregularity treated by the interceptive procedure.

It was important that the local indices should take into account any possible detrimental effects of interception as well as the benefits. The possible benefits and detriments of each treatment were listed and allocated percentage scores such that a perfect result should score 100% and a maximum detriment should score -100%. Positive marks were given as a percentage of the maximum improvement possible and negative marks as a percentage of the initial size of the criterion concerned. The overall percentage improvement or detriment was calculated by subtraction. For example: in the case of crowding treated by premolar extraction, the benefits were measured by reduction in the Irregularity Index[12] and the detriments by increased tipping and rotation of adjacent teeth, residual space and increase in the overbite and overjet.

Treatment outcome: the dental health component of IOTN was scored on the initial and final sets of casts by an independent observer who had been calibrated in the method. Initially, 69% of the children were in grades 4 and 5, which indicate a need for treatment, whereas only 42% were in these categories after the interceptive treatment. Among the children aged 9 years, 33% in Belfast moved out of grades 4 and 5 into a lower category as against

27% in Enniskillen/Omagh. The corresponding reduction among the children aged 11 years was 28% in Belfast and 24% in Enniskillen/Omagh.

As measured by the local indices, the average improvement was 71%. Treatment was completely successful in 22% of cases, deterioration occurred in 2% of cases and there was no improvement in 4% of cases. When the remaining scores were arbitrarily divided at 25% intervals, 35% showed excellent improvement, 22% good improvement, 13% moderate improvement, and 3% minimal improvement. There was little difference between age and area.

The 33% of children suitable for interception found at the initial screening is not dissimilar to the 38.6% found by Hiles[13] whose aims (to reduce or eliminate malocclusion) and methods (including simple removable appliances) were the same. Not surprisingly, the finding differs from the Burlington study of Popovich and Thompson[14] where the figures for suitable children (18% without appliances and 31% with appliances) would cover all malocclusions suitable for treatment at age 9 years. Likewise, they also differ from the Pennsylvania investigation of Freeman[15] where the ambitious aim was elimination of malocclusion.

The IOTN scores were used to determine whether the interceptive treatment was sufficient to move children out of grades 4 and 5 which indicate a need for treatment into lower grades. The fact that 69% of the children were in grades 4 and 5 at the beginning and only 42% at the end strongly supports an argument in favour of a community interceptive scheme and repudiates the reservations about IOTN as a means of scoring treatment success. It appears that IOTN and the local indices, to a large extent, were scoring the same irregularity. The outcome assessed by the local indices was equally favourable with 94% of children who completed the programme showing improvement and only 2% of children showing detrimental effects.

Thus it appears that community interceptive orthodontics has substantial benefits with few risks.

Conclusions

- Screening of children at 9 years and 11 years specifically for interceptive orthodontics can be done quickly and simply with the aid of the interception gauge.
- This screening can be combined with regular community dental inspections.
- Approximately one third of children are suitable for interceptive orthodontics.
- Children and parents are remarkably reluctant to accept offers of interceptive orthodontics and to have treatment carried out.
- The outcome of interceptive treatment is very favourable both in terms of improvement in the presenting condition and in reducing the need for subsequent treatment.
- Steps would have to be taken to educate the population in the benefits of interception before a community screening programme could make a worthwhile contribution to satisfying treatment need in the community.

* Belmark Plastics Ltd, a subsidiary of DCR Engineering 306b Newtonards Road, Belfast BT14 1HE

References

1   Adams CP. Changes in occlusion and craniofacial pattern during growth. *Eur Orthod Soc Trans* 1972: 85–96.

2   Kochhar R, Richardson A. The chronology and sequence of eruption of human permanent teeth in Northern Ireland. *Int J Paed Dent* 1998; **8**: 243–252.

3   Coulter J, Richardson A. Normal eruption of the maxillary canine quantified in three dimensions. *Eur J Orthod* 1997; **19**: 171–183.

4   Al Nimri K, Richardson A. The applicability of interceptive orthodontics in the community. *Br J Orthod* 1997; **24**: 223–228.

5   Lundy HJ, Richardson ME. Developmental changes in alignment of the lower labial segment. *Br J Orthod* 1995; **22**: 339–345.

6   Järvinen S. Incisal overjet and traumatic injuries to upper permanent incisors: A retrospective study. *Acta Odont Scand* 1978; **36**: 359–362.

7   Järvinen S. Traumatic injuries to upper permanent incisors related to age and incisal overjet: A retrospective study. *Acta Odont Scand* 1979; **37**: 335–338.

8   Landis JR and Koch GG. The measurement of observer agreement for categorical data. *Biometrics* 1977; **33**: 159–174.

9   Al Nimri K, Richardson A. Interceptive orthodontics in the real world of community dentistry. *Int J Paed Dent* (in press).

10 Ericson S, Kürol J. Early treatment of palatally erupting maxillary canines by extraction of the primary canines. *Eur J Orthod* 1988; **10**: 283–295.

11 Brook PH, Shaw WC. The development of an index of orthodontic treatment priority. *Eur J Orthod* 1989; **11**: 309–320.

12 Little RM. The irregularity index: A quantitative score of mandibular anterior alignment. *Am J Orthod* 1975; **68**: 554–563.

13 Hiles AM. Is orthodontic screening of 9-year-old children cost effective? *Br Dent J* 1985; **159**: 41–45.

14 Popovich F, Thompson GW. Evaluation of preventive and interceptive orthodontic treatment between 3 and 18 years of age. *Trans Third Int Cong Orthod* 1975: 260–281.

15 Freeman ID. Preventive and interceptive orthodontics: a critical review and the results of a clinical study. *J Prev Dent* 1977; **4**: 7–23.

Index